'A clear, simple and caring introduction to M.E. which gives the reader a good understanding of the nature of this perplexing and depleting condition. Dawes and Downing also offer much help on the road to re-establishing health.'

Leslie Kenton

Belinda Dawes received her medical training in Australia, and now runs two Christian clinics in Harley Street and Chelsea Harbour, London, for patients with post-viral syndrome. She is Assistant Medical Adviser to the M.E. Association and Medical Adviser to the M.E. Action Campaign.

Damien Downing is in private practice in York and London. He is a co-founder of the British Society for Nutritional Medicine. He is also the author of *Day Light Robbery: The Importance of Sunlight to Health*, published in 1988.

All of the patients' testimonies in this book are written in their own words.

Also by Damien Downing

Day Light Robbery: The Importance of Sunlight to Health

DR BELINDA DAWES
and
DR DAMIEN DOWNING

Why M.E.?

A guide to combating viral illness

with contributions by
DR LEO GALLAND

Grafton
An Imprint of HarperCollins*Publishers*

Grafton
An Imprint of HarperCollins*Publishers*
77–85 Fulham Palace Road,
Hammersmith, London W6 8JB

A Grafton Original 1989
9 8 7 6 5 4 3

A catalogue record for this book
is available from the British Library

ISBN 0 586 20666 3

Set in Baskerville

Printed in Great Britain by
HarperCollins Manufacturing Glasgow

Belinda dedicates this book to

Drs Leon Zimmett, Peter Barber and John Dadswell,
who believed in her and kept her going

and to her patients for their patience

Damien dedicates this book to

all the patients who helped to teach him about medicine

Acknowledgments

Belinda would like to thank all her clinic staff for their support in keeping the clinic running during her absence and her patients for bearing with it. Also thanks to Tammy for keeping her house and animals alive and Anna, Thomas and Tim for keeping her sane, and to all her friends and family who got ignored.

Finally, thanks to Damien for being such a sympathetic co-author.

Damien would like to thank all his clinic staff, in particular Barbara Hopwood, who kept everything afloat while he sank with the book.

Belinda and Damien would like to wish both their secretaries all the best in their new jobs!

Contents

Whilst we both wrote all the chapters together, the prime
responsibility for each chapter is indicated by bracketed initials.

'BE STILL AND KNOW THAT I AM GOD'

Psalm 46 v. 10

1   What is it?

M.E. stands for myalgic encephalomyelitis. This is the name now given to an illness that has been around for a number of years. In the past it has also been known as Royal Free disease, Icelandic disease, epidemic neurasthenia, post-viral fatigue syndrome, Epstein-Barr virus and many other names. This is because clusters of cases of the disease have been seen as separate entities, as outbreaks of a new virus every time. It was in the fifties, during an outbreak of the disease in Britain, that it was thought to be a relative of the polio virus and to cause a similar neurological and encephalitic disease, and therefore acquired the name myalgic encephalomyelitis.

Many doctors who are treating the condition in the 1980s feel that M.E. is a misnomer for the condition and that the term 'post-viral fatigue syndrome' is more correct. Neither of us finds this the ideal term, as it implies that there is not much more to the syndrome than fatigue. We would prefer the name 'post-viral syndrome'.

Some doctors think that we are dealing with more than one syndrome. They consider that some people are suffering from post-viral syndrome, which can linger on for months or years, and that other patients are the victims of a more sinister, organic muscular disease caused by a single highly virulent virus.

At present, the authors do not find this very convincing. It seems more likely that we are dealing with a complex of disorders, including immune dysfunction and viral opportunism. In other words, the names post-viral syndrome and M.E. describe the symptoms experienced by the patient, not the cause of the disease. It is, in fact, a diagnosis made on clinical history, on the basis of a cluster of symptoms. It is not a pathological diagnosis which can be made on the basis of, for example, a blood test or microscopic examination of a piece of tissue obtained by biopsy. Nor can it be looked up in a pathology textbook and the visible changes to tissues clearly defined.

Case Study.

Why M.E.?

Tim is a twenty-seven-year-old administrator in a charity caring
for mentally handicapped people which is run by a friend of ours. He
was a perfectly fit, healthy, energetic young man who was climbing
the career ladder at quite a rapid rate for his age. Everyone was very
impressed with his capabilities. He was a very conscientious and
bright young man who worked hard.

Suddenly in May 1986 he was struck down with flu and became
considerably unwell. After a number of weeks off work he failed to
recover. His employers, being acutely aware of post-viral syndrome
and its ramifications, sent him along to my clinic. Tim clearly had an
early but quite severe post-viral syndrome. He was bedridden and
unable to do anything for himself. He was extremely fatigued, with
bad muscle aches and pains, a lot of tummy upsets and headaches,
and was quite depressed and withdrawn.

He was also quite sceptical about the treatment, and had not come
of his own volition but on the advice of his employers. I began him on
an anti-candida diet with a number of vitamin and mineral supplements, did some nutritional tests to establish exactly the nutrients
he was lacking in and adapted his supplement programme accord-
ingly. He had a cytotoxic test and went on an elimination diet
following the results of this, and began a course of treatment of
enzyme potentiated desensitization (EPD – see p. 57).

Tim was off work for a year, and it took him almost a year with
treatment to recover fully. At the end of twelve months he was able to
return to work three days a week. When he first did this, everyone was
a little unsure as to whether he was really ready, and so he had a
further month or two at home resting.

He then returned to work again and was absolutely capable of
doing his three days a week. He rapidly increased this to five days a
week and is now working a busy full-time schedule, has a very active
social life, is functioning again entirely normally and will be married
in May 1989. (success !)

Although Tim was seen very early on in his disease, his picture is
typical of the response made by many patients to this treatment.

Almost everybody suffers from some degree of post-viral problems
at some stage in their lives. We all catch illnesses such as flu at times
and experience the after effects, when the fever and acute illness
have subsided but we feel washed out, exhausted and unable
to do much. Very few people do not experience this after a virus,

although it may last for one or two days or one or two weeks. It is also possible for this complex of symptoms that we call post-viral syndrome to occur after a serious stress other than a viral illness.

When I (DD) had my appendix removed as a medical student, I was an entirely fit young man, but for several weeks after it I felt remarkably washed out and unable to exert myself. At first I even needed to stop and rest several times on the half-mile walk from my flat to the hospital. I have also, as I have described elsewhere, seen a number of patients who have been similarly debilitated by an operation, an injury, or even a major psychological stress such as a bereavement.

Jane was a patient I (BD) saw when doing a number of clinics in Australia to attempt to help the many M.E. sufferers in that country as well.

A wife and mother, Jane was leading the typical busy lifestyle of so many people who suffer from this condition. She was involved in numerous charities and doing good works for many people. Life seemed to be going extremely well. She had a lot in her favour: a loving husband, a beautiful house, and was definitely not a neurotic housewife or a depressed middle-aged woman.

Out of the blue one afternoon, the world caught fire (well, maybe not the world, but certainly the Adelaide hills), and her house was completely obliterated. Her entire life and everything she had built up were burnt away in a single afternoon. Jane never recovered from the shock and stress of this. Her health plummeted and she began to exhibit all the symptoms of classic M.E.

Jane was the first person I had seen who had such obvious manifestations of post-viral syndrome following such an obviously non-viral cause. She led me to re-evaluate my opinion of the illness. It became quite clear to me that the symptoms of the illness are a sign of the body's inability to cope, and not symptoms of the particular cause of its failure in the first place.

I treated Jane in the same way as I have treated all the other patients I have seen with post-viral syndrome: on an anti-candida diet with vitamin and mineral supplements and excluding some foods, and EPD. She certainly began to make a dramatic improvement. Unfortunately I was only in Australia for a few months, and have not seen her for two years now. I very much hope improvement has continued and that she has been able to return to a mainstream life, as most of the other patients have.

Where then do we draw the dividing line between a normal post-viral or post-traumatic or post-operative convalescence and true post-viral syndrome? Clearly, there *is* no correct dividing line, and the decision is essentially arbitrary. We would suggest that a person needs to have been ill, suffering from the post-viral syndrome symptom complex, for at least six months before we would say that he or she had a true post-viral syndrome.

Although it is arbitrary, the distinction can be important – not least for the prognosis. It is certain that if you have had the post-viral symptoms for less than six months, your chance of spontaneous recovery is very high; but if you have had it for more than two years, particularly if it followed a clear-cut viral infection, then your chance of spontaneous recovery is unfortunately very slim. Please note that we refer to *spontaneous* recovery here. If you have had the symptoms for five years or even twenty, still do not give up. Read on and you will find that there are a number of treatments and techniques that can help you to recover from M.E.

Because M.E. is not to be found in textbooks and is a syndrome (a collection of symptoms) rather than a single disease, many doctors find it very difficult to understand and sometimes even to accept its existence. This can be a major problem for patients with post-viral syndrome. They may go to their doctor and report a spectrum of symptoms including fatigue, weakness and sleep problems, and, depending on the kind of GP they have, they can get very different responses.

More and more doctors today have heard of post-viral syndrome and are giving their patients sensible, appropriate advice – to rest, to take life quietly until they recover and so on. Most GPs appear to expect that their patients will then recover; since a GP probably sees chiefly patients with short-term cases of post-viral syndrome, this is probably sensible advice.

From our point of view, since we see many more people who have been sick for a long time and often much more profoundly sick, this is not so useful an attitude. To tell such people simply to rest until they get better would be inane because the chance of this happening is regrettably slight, and we would in effect be telling them to go away and rest for the remainder of their lives.

If your GP does not understand or recognize post-viral syndrome, then you are likely to receive one of two responses. The most common is probably that you are putting it on, it is all in your mind, and that if anything the causes are psychological. You may find yourself discussing the possible stresses in your marriage or your work, and there is probably nobody in this country who could not be found to have one or two stress factors in their life.

You may then be given one of a range of pieces of advice, from a referral to a psychiatrist to 'pull yourself together and get back to work', start exercising, or even have a baby and you will feel better. All of this is extremely counterproductive advice and likely to make the condition worse.

It is our belief that although stress can affect every aspect of your life and can certainly influence the way you handle any disease imaginable from cancer to constipation, this does not mean that such diseases are caused by stress. We suspect that very few of the complaints that are so often attributed to stress and psychological causes, and which make Valium the biggest-selling drug in the world today, are in fact psychological. Nine times out of ten there is a physical component, and identification of this is the most appropriate and effective way to treat the patient. A ruling by your doctors that your problem is psychological is really a sign that they have run out of ideas. Characterizing the problem as being in your mind rather than your body passes the buck to you and says that it is your fault that you are not getting well, not theirs. From our own experience in 'conventional' medicine, we know full well just how much pressure a doctor can experience from the endless stream of patients he or she sees, all of whom expect some sort of miraculous scientific cure. Doctors are only human, and it is no longer sensible for the patient to rely totally on the wisdom and paternalism of their GP. You need to be 'consumerist' about your doctors and to participate in deciding what treatment and what approach is most helpful for you.

The other type of response comes from a GP who is not well aware of post-viral syndrome but knows the patient to be genuine and not neurotic, and is baffled by the symptom complex. He responds by referring the patient to a succession of hospitals and specialists, looking for an answer to what appears to be an extremely obscure and unusual condition.

An example I would like to use is an imaginary patient who goes to his GP. The doctor knows the middle-aged businessman reasonably well, and knows him to be a sensible person. The patient complains that every morning when he wakes up, he has a severe headache. He also complains of disturbed concentration throughout the day, blurred vision, problems with walking in a straight line towards the end of the day, chronic indigestion and tummy ache, inability to concentrate, intermittent diarrhoea and sore red eyes. You may think I am talking about post-viral syndrome. I'm not, but please read on.

The GP who responds to this kind of symptom complex by thinking, 'Ah, headaches, poor concentration, trouble walking, he's probably got a brain tumour,' may send the patient to a neurologist. The neurologist looks for brain tumours and finds nothing, so sends the patient back to the GP. The GP thinks, 'Well, he has indigestion, intermittent diarrhoea, maybe the patient has an ulcer or bowel problem, we'll send him to a gastroenterologist.' The gastroenterologist does numerous tests and investigations and sends the patient back to the GP, having found nothing wrong with his bowel. The GP then decides that since the patient is having trouble seeing and has sore red eyes, maybe the problem is all to do with his vision, and sends the patient to an eye specialist. The eye specialist does numerous tests and investigations, with the same result: nothing wrong with his eyes. He sends the patient back to the GP.

This round of investigations and tests can cost the health service many thousands of pounds, and if anyone had bothered to ask the patient how much he was drinking, maybe the cause would have been quite clear.

I realize this is an unlikely story, and that alcohol is very easy to smell on a person. I'm just giving you a simple example of how one obvious, very common problem can have a large number of effects throughout the body, and if we don't look at the whole person we will very likely miss the explanation. We will never find the answer by looking into individual little specialities.

We are not for a moment suggesting that people with M.E. have a problem with alcohol; we are just trying to point out how a single disorder can cause problems in a large range of body systems, and how one simple step – stopping drinking – can cause remission of the symptoms throughout the whole body. Just before we leave this example, I'd like to point out that when we do tell our alcoholic to stop drinking, he is going to feel absolutely appalling for a short time. This is also true of some of the treatments we use for post-viral syndrome. Just as the alcoholic gets his DTs, so many of our patients suffer from numerous unpleasant withdrawal symptoms for a short time when we begin to treat them.

If only it were as easy to diagnose post-viral syndrome as it is to pick up chronic alcohol problems. Unfortunately, in post-viral syndrome there are no definitive tests. There are tests for some viruses, but healthy people may turn up with positive responses, and people with obvious post-viral syndrome will turn up with negative responses. So although the test is interesting and is certainly very valid from an epidemiological and virological point of view, it doesn't help us make a definitive diagnosis of who has and who has not got post-viral syndrome. It is therefore very important, if your GP is going to order one of these virological tests, that he understands the significance (or the insignificance) of the results.

In the next chapter we shall show you how a diagnosis of M.E. can be made, and look in detail at the major symptoms.

2   A diagnosis on symptoms

At present the only way to diagnose post-viral syndrome is on the symptoms and the history of the illness. The most common symptoms are, in approximate order of frequency:

Fatigue
Muscle weakness
Muscle pain
Digestive disturbances
Headache
Poor sleep patterns
Temperature-control disturbances
Depression
Lack of concentration
Muscle twitching

The only key symptom which most doctors agree is absolutely critical for a diagnosis of post-viral syndrome is that of fatigue not relieved by rest. All the other symptoms are common but not invariable. I don't think I have seen any patients who have an absolute full house of every symptom, but obviously the more symptoms you have, the more likely the diagnosis. Having said that, the symptoms need to be taken into context with a typical time course or history, and we will look more at that in a few moments.

Fatigue

Fatigue in post-viral syndrome is the key symptom, and the only one that is shared by everybody. The type of fatigue we are talking about is a brain and body fatigue where you feel as though you have just run a marathon. There is an overwhelming lack of desire to do anything other than roll over in bed and pull the covers up and ignore the world. Because of this extreme level of fatigue, many patients are thought to have personality or psychological problems. There is absolutely nothing wrong with such people's brains; the problem is that they feel totally lousy. I'm sure we can all recognize this from when we have been suffering from severe flu.

The fatigue often has a daily pattern which is common to the individual. The most common pattern, I think, is that people wake up feeling appalling and really have trouble mobilizing themselves much before lunch time. They then feel exhausted in the afternoon, but by the evening have often begun to pick up a little, so that they are able to carry on relatively normally, conversing or watching television with their friends and family. Come the time to go to bed, they are physically tired but their brain is racing and they are unable to sleep. They will often have a very disturbed night, maybe not getting into a deep sleep until six or seven in the morning, when again they sleep through till lunchtime.

This pattern is very common in the early, more acute, stages of the illness, but usually settles down as the illness progresses. It is very important in post-viral syndrome to give in to fatigue and not to try and ignore it or push it into a different time clock. To recover from this condition, you must go to bed if you want to go to bed, and stay there till way past the time you feel like getting up again.

The fatigue is also very variable. You will find most commonly that you have good days and bad days, good weeks and bad weeks, good months and bad months, and as the disease goes on, you'll probably realize that you will have good years and bad years. The reasons for this are many and varied. We have basic body rhythms which fluctuate from day to day and month to month, and this affects the baseline of how well our body copes with the illness we are suffering from. We also have times when we eat the foods which are right for us, and other occasions when we eat a lot of the foods that are wrong.

Both of these factors can contribute to the ups and downs that are experienced during the illness, but it seems that very often these variations are due to something inexplicable in the disease process itself. However, the major reason for the fluctuation (see chapter 14) is the persistent drive and determination to overdo it, so common in M.E. sufferers.

If you look at your body as a machine which is just coping, then obviously the ups and downs that everyone experiences in day-to-day life, which well people are able to manage with their built-in shock absorbers, we are less able to deal with as our coping mechanisms are already stressed to their absolute limit. Therefore life's normal daily variations affect us much more.

Muscle weakness

The muscle weakness in post-viral syndrome is extremely variable. Almost everybody suffering from post-viral syndrome has some degree of muscle weakness. I would say in the time I have been treating patients with this condition, I have probably only seen one patient who is wheelchairbound, and only two or three patients who need to be helped to walk and are really unable to do much other than sit or lie in bed. The vast majority of patients, when tested on any muscle strength test, do not show any abnormality at all. However, it is patently obvious that they are suffering from muscle weakness, and we have a very severe limitation in our medical understanding of how to test such people.

It appears that the muscle weakness in post-viral syndrome may be due to magnesium deficiency. When the body is low in magnesium, the muscle fibres are unable to relax properly. Calcium is used to make a muscle fibre contract, and people with post-viral syndrome are quite capable of contracting their muscles.

However, when it comes to being able to relax the muscle, the magnesium required to do this is not present in adequate concentration and therefore only a partial relaxation occurs.

To compensate for this, the body then contracts the muscles moving in the opposite direction to tear the muscle contraction apart and to move the particular part of the body in the opposite direction. This obviously results in some microscopic tearing within the muscles, and it is not surprising that the muscles gradually become weak and painful.

There is obviously more to the muscle weakness than just magnesium deficiency, however, and as yet we do not understand exactly what is going on.

The most common complaint in the area of muscle weakness from people with post-viral syndrome is an inability to climb stairs. Many people who are not severely affected by the condition are quite capable of walking a mile or two on the flat, going shopping for an afternoon, or spending a day pottering around the house on their feet. But faced with one flight of stairs, they are reduced to a complete blob of jelly.

It is interesting to ask why this may be the case, and I wonder if it may be due particularly to the problems with magnesium. Climbing a flight of stairs involves a rhythmic contraction and relaxation of the muscle groups in the legs on a very repetitive and quick basis, and therefore highlights the problems that the magnesium-deficient muscle has in relaxing.

A research group in Oxford has been looking at the fact that people with post-viral syndrome have a muscle metabolism which resembles that of a long-distance runner who has already run a number of miles rather than someone who has just lifted a glass of water. In these circumstances the muscle metabolism switches from 'aerobic' to 'anaerobic' functioning. The oxygen to fuel the muscles runs out, so they begin to use up glucose from stores and the bloodstream, and the body starts to produce metabolites such as lactic acid, which build up in the muscle and cause the pain that we experience on prolonged exercise. If this is so, then post-viral syndrome sufferers feel exhausted because they *are* exhausted.

There is also some evidence from muscle biopsies that there is chronic, persistent viral activity still going on in the muscles of post-viral syndrome cases. All of this points up the fact that although we don't exactly know what is going on in the muscles in such cases, there are certainly a number of very abnormal things happening there.

Until we succeed in elucidating it further and are able to offer specific advice based on a good understanding of the problem, we can only emphasize what we have learnt from the experience of many sufferers. It is important not to push your muscles, not to do any exercise, not to try and get fit, and to relax as much as possible.

Muscle pain

Muscle pain is a common symptom and probably occurs in about half the people with post-viral syndrome. A lot of people have quite mild muscle pain and, compared to all their other symptoms, really don't acknowledge it as being a symptom until it has gone. Then they say, 'Oh, wow, I didn't realize how uncomfortable I was feeling.'

Some people suffer from quite severe pain, and I have seen one teenage boy who was addicted to opiates (morphine) to control it. He required long-term, very strong painkillers for relief. This is quite unusual, and the majority of people have only a slight to mild degree of muscle pain.

The most common pains seem to be in the back muscles, followed by the muscles in the arms and legs. This pain is usually a very dull kind of ache, and is again similar to that which most people suffer from when they have an attack of flu. The other kind of muscle pain, which is probably more directly related to the viral infection, is the chest pains which a number of people suffer from. These seem to be quite different in quality from the dull back, arm and leg aches most people seem to get. The chest pains seem to be very sudden, very sharp, and often make you want to stop breathing. Fortunately, they are fairly short-lived. These can be extremely alarming, and in fact a friend and colleague of mine who suffers from them is convinced, despite her medical training, she is having a heart attack every time she has one of these, and I sympathize with her completely.

I would suggest, if you are suffering from these sorts of pains, that you do ask your doctor to investigate to make sure you do not have any underlying heart trouble. You can take comfort from the fact that many people are suffering from these types of pains and nobody seems to be coming to any harm from them. And they do settle down if you rest.

Digestive disturbances

This, again, is an extremely common problem. It is almost always due to chronic yeast infections of the gut, and is one of the symptoms, along with lack of concentration, that is extremely easy and very quick to get rid of. We will talk more about this in the section on candida and anti-candida treatment. The common problems are wind, bloating, abdominal pain and diarrhoea or constipation, or a mixture of the two.

The other common cause of colicky-type pains is food allergies, and we will discuss this further in chapter 6, but digestive problems, usually mistakenly diagnosed as irritable bowel syndrome, gastritis or hiatus hernia, are very commonly due to chronic candidiasis and food allergy.

Headache

Headache is a symptom which occurs in probably about a third of patients suffering from post-viral syndrome, and in most of these, the headache is not particularly severe. I don't think I have seen any patients who suffer from the kind of headache that would worry me or cause me to think it needs to be investigated further. Migraine is not uncommon, and has occurred in many patients who have not had migraines before, but again it is usually neither severe nor frequent. Fortunately, headache is one of the symptoms which clears very quickly with anti-candida and anti-allergy treatments.

Poor sleep patterns

As I mentioned in the section on fatigue, a poor sleep pattern is very common – typically an inability to get to sleep in the evening, broken sleep in the middle of the night, then towards early morning falling into a deep sleep, often just at the time when other people are starting to think about getting up in the morning, and then remaining in a deep sleep for several hours. If this is the pattern that your body wants, then it is really important to give in to it and not to try to get up at nine o'clock in the morning just because you think you should. If that is when your body wants to sleep, then let it. As you recover, your sleep pattern will gradually return to normal. On the other hand, I would strongly recommend that you do not think 'Oh, well, if my body doesn't want to go to sleep till 4 A.M. I will stay up and watch television until then.' Although your body may not want to go to sleep, I would still advise you to go to bed by midnight, even if you just lie there for a number of hours; your body is still resting.

As you recover, your sleep patterns will begin to recover and approach a more normal rhythm, but if you are at the stage of being ready to go back to work, you should try and negotiate with your employer some sort of flexitime so that you don't need to set an alarm in the morning. I think it is very important that you allow yourself to wake naturally as it seems to be one of the factors that really disrupts your body rhythms if you are woken unnaturally before you are ready.

A certain sign that you are overdoing it, if you have returned to work, is that when everything was going fine, all of a sudden you start not to be able to sleep and not to be able to wake up in the morning. This does not mean that you need to start setting an alarm; it means that you need to take some more time off work, you're really not ready to be doing it. You have been pushing your body into overdrive. The thing you absolutely must not do in such a situation is to start to take sleeping pills. Certainly they will allow you to sleep better, and certainly you may be able to work better, but you are beginning again the cycle of overdoing it and pushing your body beyond its ability to cope. Thus, frustrating as it may be, you need to slow back down until your body can cope with all you want to do, and you can cope with what your body wants to do.

Another common problem with sleep occurs when people who have post-viral syndrome and are plodding along just coping at work eventually – usually at my insistence – take a few months off. After the first month they very often come in complaining that they have slept almost continuously and my suggestion they stop work has in fact made them worse. This is usually not the case; what is happening is that they have been running on a little treadmill, pushing their body to its utmost limit, and when at last they do stop, their body says, 'Ah, I've been waiting for this for a long time,' and just crashes and really starts to use the rest that they are giving it. If you find that when you eventually stop, you sleep continuously, then you really should go on sleeping until you gradually wake up and start to resume some normal sleep/wake rhythms, even if this takes several months.

Just another note on sleeping pills; whilst I certainly do prescribe them occasionally, I think that with the kind of illness that we are suffering from, it is very important not to compound this by becoming addicted to sleeping pills. If you have the odd bad night when you're visiting friends, or you can't sleep on the night your next-door neighbours have their band practice, then I think there is really no reason not to take a sleeping pill. But I would suggest that under no circumstances do you take them more than three nights a week, because you are at a serious risk of becoming addicted to them psychologically if not physically.

The other sort of medication that can help sleep, and seems to be quite helpful in post-viral syndrome is anti-depressants. The one that I use most commonly with my patients is Prothiaden. Although I don't use this often, a dose of 25 mg a night, building up to 75 mg a night for a few months can often help increase the level and value of your sleep, and very often does seem to aid in recovery, but *only* if used in conjunction with a proper rest programme and the other recommendations throughout this book. Prothiaden alone is very unlikely to help in any way.

Temperature-control disturbances

Body temperature is controlled to a large degree by thyroid function and the autonomic nervous system. Both of these systems seem to be disturbed in post-viral syndrome. Thyroid function is very often disturbed in people with a whole range of environmental and allergic disorders; exactly why this is we are not sure, but it does seem to be the target for a number of auto-immune disturbances. It is important to check thyroid function. Very often, even if the function is normal, I still prescribe a low dose of thyroid hormone supplementation because there are positive levels of thyroid auto-antibodies. What causes this is the body's immune system not functioning properly. It is not under proper control and is beginning to make antibodies to its own thyroid gland, which is obviously undesirable. The body should only make antibodies to things which are foreign, not to things which are part of it. By giving a low dose of thyroid hormone, we can switch off the thyroid gland and often discourage the body from making antibodies to it, and this does seem to help a number of people with their temperature-control problems.

The most common problems people complain of are a low-grade fever throughout part of the day, or persistent coldness. If you have only persistently cold hands and feet but are otherwise normal, this is more likely to be due to a circulatory problem, and is commonly associated with magnesium deficiency rather than being a temperature-control problem. If you have a fever, this is very often due to food allergy reactions and can be controlled by eliminating those foods which your body reacts to, and I would suggest you read carefully the section on food allergies so that you can find out which foods you should be cutting out. If your whole body temperature is persistently low, then it is more likely that you have a problem with thyroid dysfunction, and you may do well with a low dose of thyroid supplementation; but first you would certainly have to see your GP or a doctor experienced in this type of medicine.

Depression

I talk a bit more about depression in the section on personality in chapter 13, but I'd certainly like to state here that depression is rarely a presenting feature of post-viral syndrome. Amongst the patients I see, most of them manage to maintain a fairly open mind and happy disposition, considering the incredible changes that have been brought about in their lives due to the illness from which they suffer. I think it is very uncommon that people are feeling ill because they are depressed; it is very much more common for them to be feeling dreadful, and therefore feeling a bit depressed because of it. Whilst I think that in some situations anti-depressant medication helps, I certainly do not advocate long-term psychiatric treatment of very many people with post-viral syndrome. A therapist who understands the dynamics within the personality that apparently cause people to succumb to chronic illnesses can be extremely valuable in aiding recovery. There are, however, therapists who think that you're depressed and if you'd just snap out of it you'd be able to function normally. This is unbelievably harmful, and if you are involved with any doctors or therapists who suggest that your post-viral syndrome is due to your attitude and you need to start pushing yourself or pulling yourself together, then you should do everything possible to remove yourself from their care.

Sarah's story

At the time, it seemed as if my illness started relatively suddenly, with an attack of flu which I seemed unable to shake off. The flu developed the night I was sitting with my dying great-aunt, a much loved person to whom I had been very close since childhood. She died that night, and early the next morning as I rang each relative to let them know, I ached and shivered all over. I returned to London and went back to work, but felt for the following month that I had not really shaken off the flu. I would wake up feeling ghastly, drag myself out of bed, have a cup of coffee and go to work. By lunch time I would start to feel better and my sore throat would disappear, but by the evening, after I had put the children to bed, I would long to collapse in bed myself and forget the pressures of the day.

Over these few weeks, together with the symptoms of flu, I also gradually began to be troubled with diarrhoea and lower abdominal pains, occasionally moving to the right and sometimes feeling like a grumbling appendix. I finally went to my GP, who examined me and thought I had a tender right kidney, so he gave me antibiotics for a kidney infection. I took these, but felt no better. The abdominal pain grew worse, so that I was frequently doubled up, and I developed a mysterious arthritic pain in my right hip, making walking painful. I returned to my GP, who sent me to see a surgeon, fearing that I had appendicitis, but the signs of acute appendicitis were lacking and I returned home again.

At this stage, I was beginning to seriously wonder what on earth could be the matter with me, and I went to see the consultant gynaecologist who had fitted my coil, thinking that perhaps I had a uterine infection. He examined me and found acute tenderness and a swelling over the region of my right fallopian tube, and diagnosed an ectopic pregnancy. I was immediately sent to hospital.

However, the hospital senior registrar could not find the swelling, and I was kept under observation for a couple of days and then sent home. The pains continued intermittently, together with the diarrhoea, and I became what felt like a human parcel between the gynaecologists and the surgeons, who were debating whether I had appendicitis or an ovarian cyst.

By this time I was starting to feel scared by all the investigations. I had never felt so ill in all my life, and yet the obvious causes had been excluded. What could possibly be going on? I decided to consult an old friend of mine, a private GP I felt I could rely on to take a comprehensive history and be thorough in his assessment. He listened to my story, did some routine blood tests and sent off a stool specimen. Surprisingly, none of these basic things had been done before. The stool specimen was promptly reported as containing three different species of amoeba, all causing amoebic dysentery. At last – a diagnosis. I felt relieved to know what the problem was, and started taking Flagyl. However, the symptoms of flu – aches and pains, shivering, sore throat and temperature – continued, together with diarrhoea and abdominal pains.

But I was reassured by speaking to two other people who had had amoebic dysentery and said that it had taken them six months to get over it. So I confidently waited for improvements, only to find myself growing weaker day by day.

At about this time, I was again admitted to hospital one night after a terrifying episode of crushing chest pain for several minutes, followed by about half an hour of irregular palpitations. Both my husband and I thought I had had a heart attack, but this was not the case. That night my pulse was very fast at 140/min, I had a temperature, and I was too weak to sit up, let alone stand up. I stayed in hospital under observation for several days, gradually improving again, and again went home, this time with a description of an anxiety state secondary to the worry over the amoebic dysentery and previous pressures of work. It was confidently predicted that six weeks off work walking amongst the early summer blossom would do the trick. So yet again I returned home and waited to get better, but found myself feeling more and more tired. The abdominal pains continued, as did the flitting aches and pains. Nothing that I did seemed to help, and I became more and more anxious about what on earth could be the matter with me. My husband took me on holiday, thinking that would put me right, but I spent most of the time too weak to walk more than a hundred yards and needing frequent rest. Swimming, once the great love of my life, had become an impossibility after the first few strokes. We returned home and I could do little more than lie on the sofa each day. Friends and colleagues kindly came to visit, and one said, 'I think you've got the same illness as a friend of mine. It's called M.E., and there was an article about it recently in the *Sunday Times*.' I mentioned this to my GP, but he pooh-poohed the idea and I forgot about it. Shortly afterwards, I became seriously depressed, and suicidal. I was admitted to a private clinic and given anti-depressants.

The next month was the most awful experience of the whole illness. The anti-depressants gave me excruciating pains, which were deemed by the staff to be caused by anxiety.

Meanwhile, the temperatures, the flitting aches and pains continued, together with the fatigue, and a sense of delirium. I could not always see properly, I frequently lost my balance or knocked things over, I found it hard to find words at times, and I felt just terribly, terribly ill. My kidneys ached; I was thirsty all the time, and producing voluminous quantities of urine.

It was at this time that I began to turn to God. I felt seized by a dreadful worry. I had always had an optimistic belief in modern medicine, that present-day doctors were good at diagnosis and treatment. Now here was I, a doctor myself, unable to find someone who could adequately diagnose and treat me. I felt, for the first time in my life, utterly helpless. I had always prided myself on being capable. No matter how awful a situation I was in, I had always been able to cope. For the first time in my life I felt completely lost and, indeed, close to death. I began to have episodes of impending doom, associated with extreme weakness. It felt as if the only firm reality was God and my relationship with Him, and I had been grasped by God and shaken by Him. It was as if He was saying, 'You've been rushing, rushing all your life, with your head down, faster, and faster. Stop, look around you, think about what really matters in your life.'

My husband, relatives and friends were very supportive throughout, but torn between the medical advice that I was physically well and simply depressed, and my own insistence that I was physically ill, and that of course I was depressed and anxious both because of the fear of what might be wrong with me, and because of my inability to do things because of the fatigue. The children were marvellous to me throughout the illness, but the worst part of it was my inability to look after them, and the fear that I might die and have to leave them motherless. I felt that I had been extremely foolhardy in taking my health so much for granted.

Towards the end of my stay in the clinic, I talked with another patient, who had got M.E. and was consulting Dr Dawes. For the second time, a lay person said to me, 'You've got M.E.'

I dragged myself into a taxi, and went to see Dr Dawes. The immense relief of being able to describe all my peculiar symptoms to someone who was already familiar with them, and said, 'I know what you've got, and I can help,' was just indescribable. I also visited Professor Mowbray, who has worked with M.E. patients for many years. Like Dr Dawes, he was familiar with all my symptoms, and was able confidently to confirm the diagnosis with the demonstration of coxsackie virus antibody complexes in my blood, and a high IgM [immunoglobulin M]. Since that time, I have had regular treatment from Dr Dawes, together with a thorough assessment of my nutritional state and advice on eating and vitamin supplements.

I returned to work, and very gradually I have started to recover, although my recovery became much faster in the second year of my illness when I finally absorbed the message that one must stay within one's physical limits, and then, paradoxically, those limits start to increase. I have had to learn to say no to people asking me to do things, something I was never able to do before. I have to budget my energy carefully through the day, and had to learn to stop immediately if I show signs of having overdone it. My husband has been particularly understanding and helpful, as he himself has experienced glandular fever and its long-term after effects.

Together with my husband and Dr Dawes, I reviewed my life and made changes to reduce the physical demands in my work and domestic life. I eventually changed my job, and we moved the children to a more local school.

It became clear in retrospect that my illness had not really started suddenly, but had slowly developed over several years of increasing fatigue, anaemia, chronic ill health, coughs and colds, etc., and exhaustion from looking after two young children, a husband and a home as well as running a busy consultant job. I had been vaguely aware of being run-down, but had simply ignored it, looking down on friends who went to bed if they had a cold – I simply assumed that ill health would go away. I now realize that getting M.E. was probably inevitable. To avert it, I probably would have had to have taken a year off work to rest and recuperate. But even then, unless I had seen a competent doctor able to diagnose and treat the amoebic dysentery and rectify the nutritional deficiencies, I was bound on a downward spiral.

I am now pulling through. I can do a full day's work, I can care for my children, and I do not have to lie down in the evenings. I can walk, but still avoid too many stairs and lifting heavy objects. I have realized that I should never return to the debilitating tempo of my previous existence, and that I have to learn to take good care of myself and to listen to my body's needs. I have learnt to enjoy today, rather than constantly rushing towards tomorrow.

The time course of the illness

The typical person who succumbs to post-viral syndrome is a high-achieving, hard-working, goal-orientated woman who does not give in easily, is certainly not kind to herself and is very much swayed by her perception of others' opinions of her. She is prone to pushing herself and is usually in a job where she is required to work quite hard, usually with a lot of overtime and long hours, and therefore is often eating a fairly poor diet.

The most common situation is that she is suffering from some sort of physical stress and at the same time an emotional stress. An example would be that she has an exam coming up, or has just had a disagreement with her boyfriend, or there has been a death in the family; and around that time, she goes down with flu or a bad cold. Very often it just takes a long time for such people to recover. Instead of being off work for two weeks with illness they return too soon, because of their hypersensitivity to others and their driving, conscientious behaviour. They then work quite hard trying to catch up, and enter a phase of not complete recovery but certainly not a serious illness, when they are never really feeling on top of things. Their health gradually begins to deteriorate, they take a number of days off because of mild coughs, colds and tummy bugs, and gradually their health declines. It is in this stage that if they recognize what is happening, they can really do something about preventing the illness from taking hold. Taking enough time off work, as sick leave and holiday leave, to recover completely from that initial immunological stress will certainly prevent the illness from progressing any further and most likely return them to complete and full health.

Unfortunately, people who are in this situation are usually not looking for health care or reading this kind of book. It is not until they again succumb to a significant viral infection which completely annihilates their coping mechanisms that they begin to look for help.

The other group of patients, whose situation is equally common, is of the same personality type, but the illness is more sudden in onset; instead of having a number of what I would call warning infections over the preceding months, they suddenly go down with a serious infection and completely fail to recover from it.

The usual time course of events, then, is that people spend several months in bed with what feels to them like acute flu. In this time, their GP and a number of other specialists are involved trying to establish what kind of illness they are suffering from, and often after a number of months they are told they are not suffering from anything and encouraged to pull themselves together.

What happens then?

After about six months, the majority of people with this condition will have completely recovered, and if you have had your illness for only a matter of weeks or months, then hopefully you'll be in this fortunate group. However, the majority of people reading this book will have had their illness for more than two years, and at that point I would say that the illness has entered a much more chronic time course and the chance of complete spontaneous recovery is fairly slim. This is really tough for me (BD) to write, and I'm sure it is tough for you to read. But it would be very dishonest of me to say, despite the fact that you may have been ill for three or four years, 'Don't worry, you will get better,' because I genuinely do not believe it, based on the people I have seen.

However, the good news is that people do not get worse, and the natural history of the illness is to remit to a degree and then follow on a fluctuating course of substandard health, but not severe illness. The even better news is that there is a lot we can do about it, and if you follow the advice and guidelines in this book, and if possible see a doctor skilled in this kind of treatment, then the chance of regaining health and recovering is extremely high.

I have treated about a thousand patients with this condition, and many of them have followed the treatment programme through for two or more years now. Of the people who are following the treatment programme, between seventy-five and eighty-five per cent are re-covering to a significant degree, certainly enough to return to work full-time and have an active social life, and are not constrained by severe dietary or lifestyle limitations – but this does take about two years of treatment to achieve.

Unfortunately, a lot of people are put off by the complexity of the treatment, and either lose faith because they are not cured within two months, or sometimes become dejected if the initial treatment makes them worse rather than better.

A number of other patients have become dejected because the regime I started them on was the same I started their friends on, and they were expecting some individualized miracle cure which was going to get them better overnight with no hiccups. This is an extremely childish and unrealistic expectation of the treatment, and the reason I start everybody on the same programme is because a large number of people who think they have post-viral syndrome are in fact suffering from chronic candidiasis, and so the first step of treatment is to eliminate candida problems. It is amazing how much this helps a number of people and it saves embarking everybody upon a very expensive and time-consuming set of investigations which many of them are not going to need.

As the treatment progresses, it becomes increasingly easy and increasingly less demanding, and is also more individualized. Doctor and patient get to know each other better, and we are able to decide upon a treatment programme that is based on individual problems and needs.

Common misdiagnoses

A number of other illnesses can resemble post-viral syndrome, and it would be impossible here to give an exhaustive list. However, the following are common problems confused with M.E.:

Chronic candidiasis
Multiple sclerosis
Hypothyroidism
Depression
Hyperventilation

Chronic candidiasis

This will be considered in the chapter on candida; the overlap between candida and post-viral syndrome is extremely large. Almost everybody I see suffering from post-viral syndrome is also suffering to a significant degree from chronic gut infection with candida, but post-viral syndrome and candida infection are not the same thing. A large number of patients are simply suffering from chronic candida overload and have no other problems, and are completely cured within months of beginning an anti-candida treatment programme. These people do not have post-viral syndrome, despite the fact that they may initially resemble the symptom picture. The distinction is important to make because if all they are suffering from is candida, and they are better in two or three months, then it is advisable for them to begin to get fit, take some exercise and approach life more positively. However, if they are suffering from post-viral syndrome and have responded quickly to the treatment, then it is very wrong for them to start attacking the world in such an aggressive manner.

Multiple sclerosis

Multiple sclerosis is a long-term neurological disease which is not always as severe as most people think. We are most aware of the people with multiple sclerosis who are severely affected, wheelchair-bound, and evoke a large amount of sympathy. However, there are many other people suffering from multiple sclerosis who perhaps don't talk about it. They have just had one or two mild attacks, and have a little weakness or visual disturbance, but are otherwise well. A number of people in this category think that they are in fact suffering from post-viral syndrome, and are misdiagnosed. They should be under the expert care of a neurologist experienced in the treatment of multiple sclerosis. There is also a great deal that allergic and environmental medicine can offer in helping the person suffering from multiple sclerosis.

Hypothyroidism

We have talked about the role of the thyroid in the section on temperature control. Hypothyroidism is a very common complaint. It causes tiredness, fatigue, dry skin and hair, heavy periods and constipation, and commonly co-exists with post-viral syndrome and other immunological problems. However, just because you have low thyroid function doesn't mean you don't have post-viral syndrome.

A number of people who think they have post-viral syndrome are really suffering from hypothyroidism, and when this is cleared up, their health returns to normal. But there is another group of patients who are hypothyroid, yet after their thyroid is treated they feel only a little better. If you have thyroid problems but don't completely recover with several months of treatment, then you are probably in the group that is suffering from M.E. and hypothyroidism concurrently, and this is quite common.

Depression

Depression is never the cause of post-viral syndrome; however, people who are feeling tired, dejected and run-down may think that they have post-viral syndrome, when they are suffering from a clinical depression. If this is the case, then therapy with an experienced psychotherapist and a course of anti-depressants will almost invariably result in recovery. It is, though, equally common for a patient with post-viral syndrome to be diagnosed as simply suffering from depression. If you are in any doubt as to whether you or your GP is making the correct diagnosis, then I would recommend you see someone who is very experienced in the treatment of post-viral syndrome and can recognize the subtle difference between the two.

Hyperventilation

Hyperventilation is overbreathing. The person doing it may be completely unaware of the fact. It also occurs quite overtly in young girls at a George Michael or Michael Jackson concert, and causes pins and needles and sometimes fainting. On the more subtle level, it causes exhaustion; usually worst after waking in the morning, and can in some cases masquerade as post viral syndrome. In other cases it can complicate a post-viral syndrome. I do not agree with those doctors who feel that there is no such illness as post-viral syndrome, and that the entire illness is due to hyperventilation. This is far too simplistic an approach; I challenge them to show me a significant success rate with a large group of patients.

I think that treating people for overbreathing is often very helpful, and if you suspect you suffer from hyperventilation, there are a number of therapists available within the NHS who would help you with this problem. Unfortunately, however, many of them will believe that hyperventilation is your only problem and there is no such thing as M.E. You may find that when they start suggesting you are 'cured', and that you should get out and start exercising, that this is very damaging to your recovery.

3 Why this book?

We felt the need to write this book in the light of the amount of publicity that post-viral syndrome has been receiving lately and the very negative emphasis of much of this. We are not aware, as authors, of any other article or book which has discussed the fact that you can get better from M.E. Having between us treated several thousand patients who are successfully recovering and getting back to work and back to living in the mainstream of life, we felt compelled to make it known that you too can recover from your post-viral syndrome.

To my knowledge, I (BD) am the only doctor in the country who treats solely post-viral syndrome, so I think I am in a position that requires I make my knowledge and experience public.

There needs to be an increase in awareness amongst the public and the medical profession that this syndrome exists, that it can be treated, and that people can get better. GPs are in the unfortunate position of never having been taught about the illness, and probably knows less about it than the patient does. We hope to reach a far wider audience by writing a book for the general public and those suffering from the condition, rather than attempting to write one for doctors on how to treat a syndrome which they are not really sure whether they believe in or not.

Who are we?

Belinda Dawes

I am Australian, and went to the Flinders Medical School in Adelaide just after it opened. Because my medical school was new, it meant that we were striving to achieve extremely high standards. It was consequently a very tough and physically and mentally demanding school to go to.

After I had done my house jobs, I moved to a children's hospital with the intention of beginning to train to become a paediatrician. Unfortunately, when I had only been there for about six months, after a series of minor viral illnesses while working a difficult roster with a lot of night duty as well as working all day, I succumbed to a glandular-fever-like illness (I am sure you all know the story). I was treated extremely well by the doctors from whom I sought advice. I don't think on any occasion did anybody suggest I may have been putting this on, or that it may have all been in my mind.

Very few doctors seemed to have much understanding of what was wrong with me, but they were at least sympathetic and encouraged me to rest, but did assure me that I would recover within a matter of months. After about six months of being off work and resting, I felt considerably better. I then decided to move to England because it seemed to me a good opportunity to make a break in my career and to change direction a little.

After about six months in Britain I tried to resume work full-time, and failed. My GP referred me to a professor in infectious diseases. This man, looking back, did not believe in post-viral syndrome, although he certainly didn't say this to me when I saw him in the clinic. He said to me that he needed to look further into my illness, and admitted me to the hospital. This seemed rather alarming to me, because I was feeling reasonably well and thought that my glandular fever illness had more or less subsided.

After a couple of days in his hospital, being in a glass box watched by nursing and medical staff twenty-four hours a day, the penny began to drop. Apparently I was being observed to work out exactly how and why I was trying to make myself ill. This was a horrifying and demoralizing experience for me, as I hadn't been treated in this way at all before. Looking back on it now, I can see that it was valuable for me to experience some of the indignation and trauma that patients are subjected to by the traditional medical profession when they are trying to seek treatment for this condition.

Needless to say, the professor and I parted company forthwith. It was only a short time before I managed to get back to work, as a part-time trainee in a practice in Yardley, in Birmingham. It was the most brilliant practice, and I will remain permanently indebted to Dr Peter Barber and his colleagues.

Dr Barber ran a committed Christian practice. At that time I was a non-Christian, so it was an interesting environment for me to work within. They also, despite being traditional doctors, were quite open to the idea of alternative medicine and to my searching for a 'cure' for post-viral syndrome. As I was increasingly preoccupied with this idea, the ground was certainly fertile for me to begin to look into alternative medicine.

During 1984 I had a very eventful year. I went to a seminar in Torquay on food allergy, and met a number of doctors from America and from this country who were treating illness through environmental, ecological, nutritional and allergic approaches. I got myself basically completely better very quickly, and at the same time David Aylin, one of the other partners, succeeded in dragging me along to Billy Graham's Birmingham mission, and this is where I became a Christian. So during this month, my life obviously underwent a large number of changes.

I began to give the patients I was seeing in Birmingham the new allergic and nutritional types of treatments that I had learnt about in Torquay. I was amazed by how successful and easy this sort of treatment was, and the patients were very kind to me. They were people with chronic illnesses who thought that there was really no hope of any recovery; they came with no expectations and they got a lot better. They were therefore far more sympathetic and far easier to cope with than some patients I see today, who come with extremely high expectations and demands.

During this time I was also asked to be the Assistant Medical Advisor to the M.E. Association, and I have been writing quite a large amount for their quarterly newsletter to encourage their membership to try to improve their health by the nutritional and allergic means which I have been describing.

In 1985 I came to London to set up a clinic specifically devoted to the nutritional and allergic treatment of post-viral syndrome and other immunological disorders.

Most of the patients I saw in the first year or two of starting my clinic are now completely well, working full-time, and leading exciting and dramatic lives. Many of the patients I saw last year are beginning to return to work, and the patients I am seeing this year are the ones who are having the hard time getting their lifestyle changed, starting their diets and beginning their treatments.

I have seen over a thousand patients with post-viral syndrome in my practice in Harley Street and Chelsea Harbour, and on several visits to Australia to treat patients there, and whilst setting up a clinic for the treatment of post-viral syndrome within the NHS at the Homoeopathic Hospital.

The treatment is extremely successful, and it is also very demanding.

One of the main complaints from patients now is that the treatment is too hard. The treatment is obviously difficult. It is our lifestyles that made us ill in the first place, therefore it is our lifestyles that need to change, and if we are going to change our lifestyles, then of course it is going to be hard.

A graph I draw for every patient who comes to see me on their first visit describes the aims and the expectations of this treatment, and is worth going through again. The picture of how quickly you are likely to recover whilst doing this treatment is basically this:

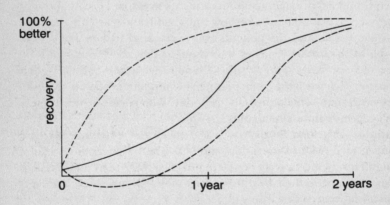

The unbroken line is the *average* time course of how long it takes to recover. At nought is when you first come and start the treatment; you are then at the level of no recovery. You gradually improve for about a year, and then at about the one-year mark things seem to improve quite dramatically. After about two years, the improvement tails off at about your previous level of health. Sometimes better, sometimes not as good, but certainly within that area.

The dotted lines either side represent the range of responses. In other words, some people recover extremely quickly; within three or four months they are almost better, then they just go on and improve and reach a plateau much quicker. Other people get worse for the first few months, but then they go on and improve. After a few months of trauma they eventually recover to the same level as everybody else.

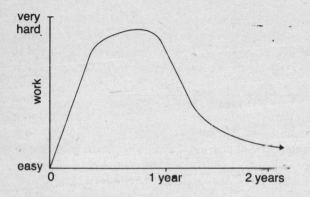

The second picture I have drawn here is the amount of work you need to do. By work, I mean changing your diet, changing your lifestyle and changing your thought patterns and attitudes. Things get very tough very quickly, and then for the next few months they go on getting even tougher. It stays pretty tough for six to twelve months and then gradually the difficulty decreases. That means that you no longer need to stick to a diet, you no longer need to watch what you eat, you no longer need to take loads of vitamin and mineral supplements and you no longer need consciously to change your attitudes. I don't mean you can go back to your old ways, but the necessary changes will be ingrained and your thinking will be different.

The third picture (overleaf) is the cost of the treatment in our clinic. In the initial sessions, the number of biochemical and allergic profiles we do and the vitamin C infusions we give to boost the patient's immune system are relatively expensive, so, unfortunately, the cost is all incurred in about the first four to six weeks. After that the treatment is relatively cheap, at a total cost of a couple of hundred pounds a year. I know it is not free, but to be back working and earning money, this is not expensive.

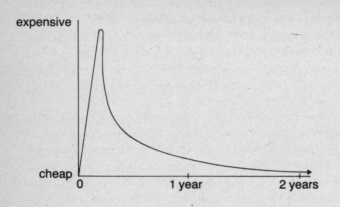

As well as being interested in post-viral syndrome, I am a trustee of United Response, a Christian charity for residential care of people with mental handicap. I am also a patron of the Suzy Lamplugh Trust. Suzy was an estate agent who vanished during her work in July of 1987. Her mother has set up a trust to promote awareness of women in the workplace and to encourage research and education in the area of the safety of women at work. And I am a home group leader in the church that my staff and I attend.

Damien Downing

In a way, I have been practising medicine since I was thirteen. At that time, we lived in Nigeria, and my mother helped to run a mission hospital. There was only one doctor, and sometimes there were many urgent operations such as Caesarean sections to be performed every day. In the school holidays, I went there to help, and became quite accustomed to scrubbing up for operations and holding a pair of forceps or a retractor while a baby was delivered or an internal haemorrhage repaired. I eventually formalized this arrangement by studying medicine at Guy's Hospital, and practised in conventional medicine in the National Health Service for several years. But then, as a result of the illness of somebody very close to me being cured by acupuncture, I became interested in the subject and took a qualification in it. After working abroad for three years to raise the money to leave the NHS I came back and set up as an independent practitioner in acupuncture. The following two years were an exciting time medically, and many people got well who had previously not been helped by ordinary medicine. On the other hand, a number did not respond. When, after about a year of practising acupuncture, it was suggested to me by two patients at once that food allergy might have something to do with their problems, I started to experiment in this field.

The results were immediately dramatic, and I became hooked on the use of food allergy in treatment. From there it seemed only a small and natural step into the use of nutrition as a therapy. At that time there were no opportunities to be taught formally about these methods in Britain, and I had to go to the USA on several occasions to study. Since then, I have discovered more and more exciting techniques that can be used to benefit patients who have not been helped at all by orthodox medicine. These days, I wonder whether I should invoke the patronage of St Jude and rename my practice 'the clinic for hopeless cases'.

Over the past few years, M.E. has become a large and challenging part of my practice, as I am sure it has for many other practitioners of this and similar forms of medicine. Now we are confident that we know enough to help the large majority of cases, but I have to admit that it has been a learning experience for me as well as for the patients. They have not only had to accept being guinea pigs to some extent, they have also had to help me, with their insights and their ideas, to help them.

4   You are out of balance

As well as asking 'Why me?' the most common question people suffering from post-viral syndrome seem to ask is, 'What went wrong; why did I get this diabolical illness?' The principles of orthodox medicine, which assume that every disease has a single cause and a single treatment, don't work in post-viral syndrome.

M.E. is a problem of whole body overload, as a result of which we are highly susceptible to anything which is passing. We talked about this when we discussed the definition of M.E. and talked about our bodies' immunity versus the virulence of the bug we are encountering. In post-viral syndrome the immune system's capacity appears to be in some way diminished. The fact that we are unable to measure this is medicine's failing, not the patient's. In conceptual terms, if the body and its immune defences are not working properly, then something *must* be wrong. In a very simplistic manner you can say that the body is either suffering from too much of something or too little of something.

I think it is very helpful to look at the body in this way as it enables us to escape the constraints of the single cause, single effect model of

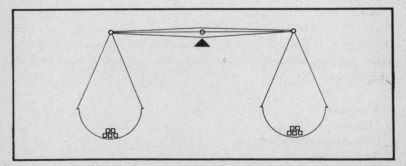

Figure 1   You are in balance: neither too much nor too little of anything.

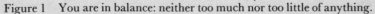

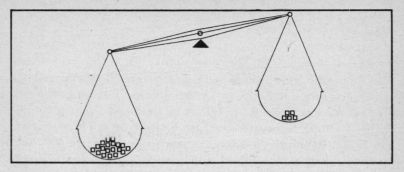

Figure 2 The body is way out of balance. Too much of a number of things and too little of a number of other things

illness and start looking at the body as a whole, and at all the things that affect it.

This concept of illness was first discussed, to my knowledge, by Dr Sidney Baker, who is a very wise doctor of allergic and environmental medicine in Newhaven, Connecticut. If we look at the large pan, the things we have too much of, this contains:

Allergies
Candida
Parasites
Toxins
Pollution
Stress
Infections
Work

If you look at the pan that is too small and contains too little for balancing the demands of the other side, this pan should contain adequate amounts of:

Vitamins
Minerals
Oils and fatty acids
Amino acids
Oxygen/carbon dioxide

Rest
Love
Self-esteem

This view of our body is simplified but extremely helpful. We will talk about allergies, candida, toxins, stress, infections, vitamins, minerals, oils, essential fatty acids, amino acids, rest and love, in specific chapters devoted to these topics. By reading this book, I hope that you will be able to unload the heavy side and load up the light side, and gradually bring your body back into balance.

Another way of looking at the problem of your body being over-loaded and causing post-viral syndrome is to consider a ship sailing – perhaps around the coast of the Med, where it needs to stop at a number of ports to load and unload cargo (Figure 3).

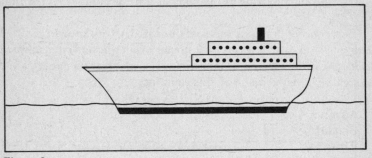

Figure 3

As the ship stops at its various ports it is getting heavier and heavier, with more and more boxes of cargo being placed upon it (Figure 4). Suddenly, between ports, for no good reason, the ship

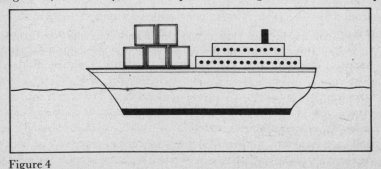

Figure 4

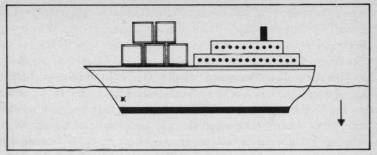

Figure 5

strikes a small object under the water, and a tiny hole is pierced in the hull (Figure 5).

Because of this small hole, the ship begins to sink. There are two ways of rescuing the ship. We can either send down the divers, which is great if we have a diving team, or we can throw off the cargo so that the hole comes above the water line (Figure 6).

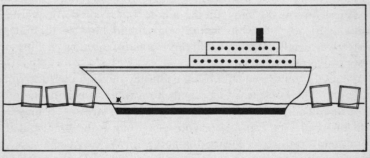

Figure 6

Having unloaded the cargo, the ship is now able to sail happily around, doing a large number of activities. Despite the hole in its hull it is perfectly stable, so long as it doesn't get overloaded again.

This analogy of the ship sailing around, collecting more and more boxes of cargo, is very illustrative of the kind of person that gets post-viral syndrome. They sail through life collecting more and more stresses and loads on their body. Each of these boxes can represent vitamin and mineral deficiencies, lack of rest, poor diet, increasing amounts of food allergies, candida overload, chemical toxicity and pollution, and any number of stresses we care to place on our bodies. Again, each of these will be discussed in a separate section of the book.

When the person succumbs to an intercurrent viral infection (like the small hole in the ship), it is not the particular virus that is the problem, it is just that a small virus has created a small hole in an otherwise overloaded person and the person, like the ship, begins to sink. Like the ship, we have several alternatives in treatment. Just as we could mend the hole in the ship by sending down divers, we could mend the hole in the person if we knew how to kill viruses. Unfortunately, there are no successful specific anti-viral treatments, and, besides, we are not sure which particular virus, if any, is causing this syndrome, so it is obviously quite impossible to mend this hole. However, just as we can unload the ship, we can unload our body from all the various stresses. This is the aim of treatment: to rebalance your body's ability to cope with the stresses it is under, by bringing the hole above the water line and unloading some of the burdens your body is carrying around.

By reading the chapters which follow, we hope that you will unload your body and regain health and vitality. Your body will still have a weakness, just as the ship still has a hole, but if you don't overdo it, don't overload your ship again, you should be able to function perfectly normally. We hope that this is some of the most encouraging news you have read so far.

We invite you to join with us on a journey through the subsequent chapters of this book, learning exactly how, when, why and where you need to unload your body from your particular stresses. It may be a difficult road. We can assure you it is going to be long, but it is absolutely worthwhile. Please don't give up. We can also assure you that many hundreds of people, including myself (BD), have followed this path and gradually unloaded their bodies, just as sailors have unloaded the ship, and are now working and functioning happily and healthily without their overloaded cargo.

5   Immune dysfunction

The human brain is said to be the most complex organic system in the world. But there is another system that is just as complex. Until recently, we knew nothing about it because it is not so visible; it does not occupy a single space in the body but is spread throughout all our tissues. This is the immune system. In this chapter we shall be looking at what the immune system is, what it does, and its importance for M.E. sufferers.

There are several similarities between the immune system and the brain. They both have the function of identifying external features of the environment and reacting to them. They both, therefore, have the ability to learn and remember. As we are now coming to appreciate, they are also very closely interconnected with each other.

The central purpose of the immune system – so far as we think we understand it – is to discriminate between those molecules that should be in the body and those which should not, and to dispose of the latter. In other words, it identifies what is 'self' and what is 'not-self'.

A newborn baby has a very undeveloped immune system, but fortunately, for the first six months of life the baby is protected by antibodies and other factors it has acquired from its mother. By the time these are out of its bloodstream its own immune system should be up and running.

During these early stages of development, the immune system is chiefly learning what molecules are 'self', and remembering not to attack them. It then knows that any other molecules which it identifies are likely to be 'not-self', and it views them with suspicion. With a minimum of persuasion, it will develop antibodies against such a molecule, and eliminate it from the body.

There is a fine balance in this, and there are two major things that can go wrong. First, through overstimulation and a variety of other stresses, the immune system can become overactive. This tends to lead to food allergies and chronic symptoms caused by reactions to relatively normal components of the environment. On the other hand, if the immune system becomes underactive, perhaps due to a lack of the essential nutrients that it requires for proper functioning, or general exhaustion, then the body can become vulnerable to infections, and possibly even to diseases such as cancer.

Consider a simple case of measles, because this is a straightforward example of normal functioning by the immune system. Assuming that you have never before been exposed to measles, the first time your body encounters it, it is required to make antibodies against the measles virus from nothing. This takes a few days, starting when the virus first starts to multiply within the body. At this stage, the problem is likely to be localized to the upper respiratory tract, and the symptoms are going to be snuffles and sneezes and sore itchy eyes.

Gradually, the virus starts to spread, first down the respiratory tract and into the lungs, and then throughout the body. At the same time, your immune system is racing to develop antibodies against the virus. When it finally does so, it releases these antibodies in large numbers throughout the system. They attack and latch on to measles viruses, and form into clumps known as immune complexes.

Wherever one of these immune complexes is deposited in the body, there is a reaction as other cells of the immune system gather round and attempt to digest the immune complex and eliminate it from the system. This produces the characteristic spots of measles – which are not just something that happens on the skin, they are spread throughout every tissue of the body. Measles spots, therefore, are not so much evidence of the disease as a sign that the body has won a victory over the disease.

When this has been achieved and the measles virus has therefore been eliminated from the system, the body still has the starting block for making antibodies against measles. If there is no use for that antibody then production of it will shut down, and the amount circulating in the bloodstream will gradually decline. If, in years to come, the body is again exposed to measles, then it can quickly mount a response, without having to learn how to manufacture that particular antibody again, but it does not waste energy by keeping large numbers of antibodies around unused.

The commonest abnormality of this system is a food allergy. This is a very different pattern of functioning from the measles example, and one that has a great deal to do with the development of chronic immune malfunctions. There are a number of ways that a food allergy can develop, and we shall be looking at these in a moment. There are certain common features, though.

The body is exposed to an antigen (something it wants to fight), which is most typically a common food such as wheat or milk (but may well be several of them). As a result of this exposure, the immune system develops antibodies against the food. This exposure can carry on for years, instead of being over and done with in a couple of weeks, as in the case of measles or most other infections. The body, therefore, continues to produce antibodies against the food for as long as the exposure goes on. The effect is much like having a chronic infection for months or even years. It leads to a depletion of the body's resources in general, with secondary consequences from this depletion, as well as causing symptoms directly through the allergy itself. However, the sufferer often does not make the connection between feeling unwell and eating the causative food.

Food allergies are important because they are very common; thirty per cent of people asked in a British survey, and forty per cent in an American one, said that they had an unpleasant reaction to certain foods and therefore avoided them. There are unquestionably many more people who have reactions to foods but are unaware of them.

This is significant to M.E. sufferers for two reasons. First, because a large proportion of people with M.E., when their past history is examined in detail, turn out to have had food allergies for nearly all their lives, and to have had a degree of ill health as a result, which they have done their best to ignore.

Second, almost everybody that we see with M.E. has food allergies *now*, and they are playing a major part in the disease process of M.E. It is worthwhile, therefore, going back and looking at the origins of these problems. We are not saying M.E. is caused by food allergy, but that most people have some minor food allergies causing minor problems. If the body becomes weakened by an illness such as M.E., any factor which is further burdening the body should be dealt with to enable the system to recover.

The immune system of the newborn child is rather like a computer waiting to be programmed. The information to achieve this programming comes largely from the mother's immune system, through the breast milk. The milk, and particularly the colostrum that comes in in the first couple of days of breast-feeding, contains a very high number of antibodies known as secretory immunoglobulin A (sIgA) antibodies.

These seed into the lining of the baby's intestine and programme the rich patches of immune areas in the gut with the necessary information. They teach the immune system that there are certain proteins and other components of the incoming food to which it should not respond, and others to which it should respond. Without this information, the child's system will inevitably make mistakes and react inappropriately.

If a baby is not breast-fed, it loses its one and only chance to acquire this information and is much more likely to develop allergies. Plenty of people (myself included) recover from this and go on to live perfectly normal lives. But it is a general truth that while the body can nearly always recover from one thing going wrong, it may find it impossible to get over two or three things going wrong on top of each other. M.E. is in many cases a very good example of this; we simply have a large number of factors all going wrong at once and the body's defences eventually fail.

It can happen, of course, that a child is born with its immune system already programmed to react with allergies. That is to say, it inherits the allergy from one or both of its parents. This plays a large part in allergies of the asthma/eczema/hayfever type; if both parents have allergies of this type, the child has roughly an eighty per cent chance of suffering too. But it also seems to occur with food allergies, although the pattern is less well understood as yet. It is also common for food allergies to develop when a baby is weaned, or started on cow's milk.

Presumably this presents more unknown protein to the digestive system than it can handle all at once, and large amounts of this protein find their way into the bloodstream, where they naturally trigger off an allergic reaction. Since, if the problem goes unidentified, the child will continue to consume milk for years, the symptoms will also carry on. The reaction may cause, for example, colic, stuffy nose and behaviour problems in the baby, tummy aches and headaches in the school-age child, and then migraine and arthritis in the adult.

This pattern of an overload of the system leading to the development of allergies can also occur at any time throughout life. For example, the foods to which people most commonly develop allergies are those which they eat most frequently. In our society this means foods such as wheat, milk, eggs, and nowadays colourings and additives. In other societies this could mean rice, nuts, beans, and so on. It is not clear whether frequent exposure to foods in this manner is itself a sufficient insult to the system to trigger reactions, or whether it simply makes it more likely that the foods are in the system when something else goes wrong, such as an infection. Either way, the effect is the same.

Breast milk is also important because it encourages the growth of the normal organisms that inhabit the gut. These will be discussed more in another chapter, but here we should look at their importance for digestion, and for food allergies. The normal flora of the gut has a number of vital roles to play. It assists in the digestion of the foods we eat, breaking down proteins and carbohydrates so that they can be more easily absorbed. This has the consequence of reducing the amount of protein around to which the body can react with an allergy. The organisms also manufacture more vitamins from the food that we eat, and make these available to the body.

Infection can lead to the development of allergies in a couple of ways. When an infection of the stomach or bowel occurs, this can kill off the normal flora and eliminate that line of defence; or, much more commonly, the antibiotics used to treat the original infection will just kill off everything in sight, good and bad. The infection may also interfere with the normal production of digestive juices, which break down proteins, including bacteria and viruses, and protect the body against infections of this very sort. The gut therefore becomes even more vulnerable to such infections. As a result of the overgrowth of hostile organisms, and of the lack of the normal protective ones, the bowel may become inflamed and more porous, allowing protein into the bloodstream. The infection can then spread from the bowel into the whole body, and food allergens can pass across into the bloodstream and trigger the immune system to produce antibodies.

A good example of this, and one which most doctors working in the field will easily recognize, is that of a woman who went to India in her early twenties, living on a limited income and therefore eating badly, and suffered a severe attack of gastroenteritis. During the recovery phase she could not face solid food, and so lived almost entirely on milk and milky foods. By the time she came home she had a chronic irritable bowel syndrome, and in fact she did not recover her strength or her health for a number of years. The gastroenteritis had stripped the lining of her bowel; when she poured milk on to it, it was absorbed into the bloodstream, and her immune system immediately set up a reaction to it. This led to the chronic bowel problem, plus a seriously impaired digestive system which caused her to become deficient in quite a few nutrients. As a result, she was permanently fatigued and run-down, and it only took a relatively minor further infection to turn her problem into full-scale M.E.

When someone has a food allergy, it seems that the body is too involved in reacting to and trying to eliminate that food to be able to absorb the nutrition from it. He or she is quite likely therefore to develop a deficiency of the vitamins or other nutrients for which that food is the source. If, as is very often the case in M.E., there is also a disturbance of the organisms in the bowel, this provides another factor which deprives the body of vitamins, and a deficiency becomes even more probable.

The need to respond to an infection mobilizes the immune system and puts it on the defensive. It rapidly develops antibodies to any suspicious protein at this time. If there is food protein – as in the case cited there was quite a lot of milk protein in the bloodstream – then it is likely to undergo what is known as an 'innocent bystander effect', and become the target of a new antibody even though it is not responsible for the infection. Once this reaction to a food is established, it is often kept active by eating the food regularly. As the body tries to adapt to this new state of affairs, this can even lead to addiction and a feeling of need for regular doses of the food every day. This, of course, serves only to 'irritate' further and stimulate the immune system, and it becomes quite likely that other reactions to foods will develop.

In such a case it is reasonable to say that the immune system is overactive. This is likely to show on testing of, for example, the ratio between different types of T-cells in the body. T-cells, which are a particular type of white blood cell, are a major means by which the body regulates the level of activity of the immune system. They are divided into T-helpers, which stimulate the immune system to attack antigens, and T-suppressors, which retard and control this attack. There is a normal healthy ratio of helpers to suppressors, which is around two to one or just under. A ratio higher than this indicates an overactive immune system, and a lower ratio indicates an under-active one.

There are some major medical disorders which affect the T-cell ratio in a big way, but these need not concern us now. One of them, of course, is AIDS, in which the virus specifically attacks the T-helpers. In M.E. it is very common to find a lowered helper to suppressor ratio; however, it is equally or slightly more common to find an elevated ratio. An abnormality in either direction is possible but a normal result is quite rare. The reasons for this require a little bit of explanation.

First, people with M.E. have very often had problems with aller-gies, particularly hidden food allergies, before they develop the full syndrome. This may have arisen as a result of infection, or for any other reason. They may even have been born with the tendency. Whatever the cause, these reactions lead to an overstimulation of the immune system. It reacts to more and more things, and gradually depletes the body of nutrients as it uses them up in these reactions.

At some stage it is likely that this overactivity and gradual de-pletion will reach a point where the body can no longer sustain the activity. This is a recognized pattern of events in physiology in general, and was well described by Hans Selye in his general theory of adaptation. This explains, in several stages, what happens when an organism is required to adapt to a stress. At first, it pulls out all the stops and responds satisfactorily, becoming overactive in the process.

Eventually, however, it reaches a stage of exhaustion, and the mechanisms in question more or less shut down. We have all experi-enced something similar to this when we have worked flat out to respond to a crisis or to reach a goal or deadline, and then collapsed afterwards and taken days or weeks to recover. In the mechanisms we are describing here, however, the collapse is normally determined by physiological factors, not by the mind.

If and when such a collapse occurs, the body immediately becomes vulnerable to a number of problems. The T-helper to suppressor ratio drops to well under the two-to-one mark, and the immune system becomes underactive and inefficient.

However, it is unlikely to have got rid of its allergies, so what little functioning there is in the immune system is still involved in reacting inappropriately to foods. This means there are fewer resources left over for responding to infections. M.E., of course, is very often triggered by a virus or similar infection, and it may well be this very infection that is the last straw, leading to partial collapse of the immune system. The body becomes scarcely able to cope with this or other infections, and further chronic infections with viruses and fungi become highly probable.

We are then left with the bizarre circumstance of a double imbalance of the immune system. While it has been overactive it has learnt to react to a number of foods and other non-threatening components of the environment.

Now that it has become underactive it continues to react to these, but is less capable of reacting to infections. This means that treatment measures which aim simply to raise the level of activity of the immune system, while they help the body to cope with its infective problems, will be likely to make the food allergies worse.

Measures that suppress the immune system, on the other hand, would lay the body open to infections to an even greater extent, while achieving little for the food allergies. What is necessary is a double-pronged approach which controls the allergies while stimulating the immune system's ability to respond to infections and other attacks from outside or inside. In subsequent chapters we shall see how this can be achieved.

At the beginning of this chapter we stated that in its complexity and in its role the immune system was strikingly similar to the brain. A further aspect of this similarity is that they are both particularly vulnerable to disorders of nutrition. As anybody who has worked with computers will confirm, the more complex a system is, the more things can go wrong with it. So it is with both the nervous and immune systems.

For the immune system to respond successfully to an outside stimulus, such as the presence of an antigen, a large number of stages have to be gone through. The antigen has to be discovered and its presence notified to the rest of the immune system. If appropriate, the body has to design and build an antibody against it, and then produce it in large numbers. The same complexity holds for other responses, such as that required for desensitization. Each step of immune activity is in itself complex, requires the correct balance of conflicting factors, and also consumes a considerable amount of energy. As a consequence, the immune system is vulnerable to a variety of things going wrong, and one of the commonest and most documented areas of such problems is nutrition. It has now been demonstrated by a large number of scientific experiments that a deficiency of any one of the vitamins, minerals, amino acids and essential fatty acids necessary to the body's functioning can lead to a disorder of the immune system – either overactivity or underactivity. Since people with M.E. already have both a disorder of the immune system and very probably some disorder of nutrition as well, it is clear that they can be heading for a downward spiral, with nutritional and immune problems complicating each other in a self-perpetuating system.

In subsequent chapters, particularly Chapter 8, we shall see how specifically targeted and adjusted nutritional therapy can be used to regulate the immune system of M.E. sufferers, and how it becomes an important part in the overall treatment regime.

Quite apart from the similarities between the immune system and the nervous system, they are closely interconnected and influence each other all the time. The whole of the immune system – the liver and spleen, the regional lymph glands in the armpits, groin and neck, and all the immune tissues elsewhere – is well supplied with nerves, and constantly receives regulatory signals down these nerves.

There is also an indirect means of regulation by the nervous system, through the endocrine system. The endocrine glands, such as thyroid, adrenal and the sexual organs, are subject to neural control both directly through the nerves that run into them, and through the hormones produced by the anterior pituitary gland at the base of the brain. These hormones in turn influence every cell in the body, stimulating, suppressing or modifying their activity.

The cells of the immune system are no exception to this. We have known for some time that the immune functioning can be altered by the levels of hormones in the blood – including the stress hormones produced by the adrenal, and the sexual hormones, most typically during the female menstrual cycle. There is also a traffic in the opposite direction. The immune system sends signals to the nervous system along the same nerves, feeding back information on how the immune functions are performing.

The brain and nervous system can also be influenced by the presence of immune complexes (combinations of antibodies and antigens), which are likely to reach it through the bloodstream both in the case of infections and that of allergies. These can modify the functioning of the brain, and indeed the mind, in a number of ways.

They may provide mild stimulatory or depressant influences on the level of activity of various groups of nerves. They can even seriously disorganize the brain and lead to problems such as schizophrenia or epilepsy. Naturally, the more extreme forms of dysfunction are less common than the mild forms.

A typical pattern of problems would be that the presence of immune complexes in the brain produces symptoms such as chronic fatigue, lack of energy and general malaise. Reactions to specific foods would then cause, on top of this, further symptoms such as attacks of depression or severe headaches.

We already know that our state of mind and our mood can dramatically influence the functioning of the immune system, as well as the digestive system, and probably every other cell in our bodies. Experiences such as bereavement can cause a temporary collapse of the immune system, during which it has been shown that the immune response to stimuli can be depressed, and during which it is possible for long-term problems such as allergies to arise. In other words, we are looking at yet another self-sustaining vicious cycle of interactions which can operate to keep a sufferer ill.

All hope is not lost however; these problems are treatable. In order to do so, though, we need knowledge, skill, and a complex multi-factorial approach. For example, it may be necessary to combine desensitization, nutrition and psychotherapy.

Desensitization will serve to bring the allergies under control, and to clear the immune complexes from the brain. Nutrition can be used to improve the functioning of the brain, to raise or regulate mood and emotional status and to feed the immune system.

We can even, if it is completely necessary, use drugs such as anti-depressants to do the same thing. But it may certainly be necessary to use forms of psychotherapy, or related measures, in which people are able to express their feelings more. As their own attitudes and problems change their immune function improves.

Another important and effective method of outside immune control that one of us is using in many patients is that of prayer. This is discussed in more detail in another chapter.

In many ways, M.E. is not a sudden plague that descends on a hapless sufferer so much as the point when a set of problems reaches what in nuclear physics is known as critical mass: when a destructive interaction becomes inevitable. In other words, the multiple malfunctions that make up M.E. do not descend upon you out of the blue. They have been quietly developing, in most cases, for months, years, maybe even decades. I hope this chapter has helped you to understand how a minor event in the immune system can set up ripples which spread throughout the whole body, and through every system, and build up to a tidal wave. In subsequent chapters we are going to discuss in detail what can be done to treat these problems.

6   Food allergies

Food allergy is not the cause of M.E. or post-viral syndrome, but it is an important component of it. In fact, allergies come into the categories of <u>both cause and effect</u>, and are another box of cargo on our sinking ship. The majority of M.E. patients are totally unaware of their food-allergy problems.

In the previous chapter we discussed a number of aspects of the immune system and its importance in post-viral syndrome. From this it is clear that in many cases long-term hidden food allergies precede the development of post-viral syndrome, often by a number of years. Food allergies are among the first things that go wrong with the immune system – in fact, they create the fertile soil into which the seed of the virus or other trigger to M.E. then falls. However, when M.E. has developed, it is clear that the immune system becomes even more disordered, and substantially worse allergies are likely to develop. In these circumstances, the allergy is clearly an effect of the M.E.

In this chapter we will look first at the various patterns of allergy that can be identified, then at methods of diagnosis, and finally at the treatments which are available for the problem.

Patterns of allergy

To most orthodox doctors, even nowadays, allergy has a very narrow and precise meaning. It refers to the group of reactions that we call atopic allergy. To nutritional physicians, and to all of us who believe that post-viral syndrome is treatable, allergy has a much wider meaning. The atopic allergies include such disorders as asthma, eczema, hayfever, perennial rhinitis (or vasomotor rhinitis), conjunctivitis and urticaria. These syndromes are in many ways interchangeable, in that an individual may suffer from asthma at one stage during his or her life, and eczema or hayfever at another time. They also have in common the presence of high levels of a particular type of antibody, known as IgE antibodies, in the bloodstream. They also fall into a category known as fixed allergies. This means that whenever one is exposed to the allergen, there is a reaction. For instance, hayfever sufferers experience their symptoms every summer and a cat-allergic person will sneeze almost every time he is with a cat. The large majority of allergies are very different from this in their pattern, as we shall see.

The importance of the atopic allergies in a post-viral syndrome is unique. The two problems appear to be mutually exclusive. People who have asthma or other atopic reactions seem to lose them when they develop post-viral syndrome. Often, when the post-viral syndrome is successfully treated, the atopic reactions come back, which may lead one to believe that the treatment is ineffective. In fact, the recurrence of these allergies is a demonstration that the M.E. *is* being treated.

Between them, the authors cannot recollect a single case of some-body who had a full post-viral syndrome and also concurrently suffered from a full-blown atopic allergy. However, after treating several thousand patients, we have often seen atopic allergies return during successful treatment.

Many non-atopic allergies, which constitute the large majority of reactions, fall into the category known as masked allergies, in which addiction plays an important part. The general theory of adaptation developed by Hans Selye, which we discussed in the previous chapter, appears to explain many aspects of these reactions. When the body is constantly exposed to allergens, it tends to adapt and comes to treat the presence of the allergen in the bloodstream as being normality. As a result, provided that the level of allergens is kept more or less constant, the symptoms are kept to a minimum by the body. A major change in the level of allergens, however, will provoke symptoms, and these are the same whether the change is an increase or a decrease. An increase, or an overdose effect, produces the same symptoms as a decrease, or withdrawal. To stay comparatively well, allergens need to be kept at a level which the body will tolerate. This is one of the reasons why most M.E. patients are either over- or undereaters, and thus over- or underweight.

From the very choice of words here, it is clear that we are talking about an addiction, and it is certainly true that people with this sort of allergy tend to crave the foods to which they react, or at least to regard them as a normal, regular part of their diet.

When we treat them for these problems, if the treatment entails cutting the allergen out, then it is highly likely that a period of withdrawal symptoms will ensue. We often have to do battle with patients to convince them to try cutting out their favourite foods.

All the time that this is going on, there is constant stress on the body. Although there may be no acute symptoms, there are very likely to be chronic ones, which will very probably include the core symptoms of allergy.

These are symptoms such as fatigue, drowsiness during the day, bloated stomach after food, sensation of pressure in the head, headaches, impaired concentration or memory, and even inability to focus. Apart from these, there is also a vast range of other symptoms which may occur, from diarrhoea to depression, and from backache to boils. People with these problems, even if they do not have post-viral syndrome, have often become so used to living with the symptoms that they have forgotten what it is like to be well. It is only when we clear the allergens out of the body and the withdrawal symptoms have passed that they can hope to improve. It is often necessary to eliminate all the allergens at once for the system to improve. Very often people will try a week or two without a particular food – say, milk or wheat – and reintroduce it with no effect. Unfortunately, we cannot conclude that this means no food allergy. It is necessary to try to eliminate all offenders for a week or two and then try reintroducing them one at a time, and this can be quite complicated.

In terms of the theory of adaptation, this is when the body is, more or less, withstanding the strain of these allergies, although at a price. After a period of some years, it may happen that the adaptation will break down, the body will no longer cope with the allergens, the patient will become substantially more generally ill, the addictions will get more unstable and the reactions to foods more overt. If the symptoms during the adapted phase were relatively mild, it may only be at this stage that the patient seeks treatment.

A few years ago a lot of media attention was given to what was termed the total allergy syndrome. Although this exists, it is unquestionably rare; there cannot be as many as a hundred sufferers in this country. There must be, on the other hand, a number of people who at that time strongly suspected that they had the syndrome, but who have now tentatively rediagnosed themselves as having post-viral syndrome. In the majority of cases, the rediagnosis will be the correct one.

Both diseases can make you feel extremely ill, and the symptoms may be very similar, but it is important to achieve a correct diagnosis because the treatments are quite different. Although it can be just as crippling, M.E. is definitely the more treatable of the two. It can mimic total allergy syndrome, because the patient may react to so many foods. However, in M.E. this is due not only to allergy but also to the presence of candida in the bowel, which can cause reactions to carbohydrates and yeast products.

There is a further, pseudoallergic, problem which can become confused with both of the above diagnoses, and this is severe chemical sensitivity. People with this problem tend to get symptoms not only from exhaust fumes but also tobacco smoke, scents, deodorants, household chemicals, and even the formaldehyde and other chemicals used as adhesives for carpets and the dressing of new clothes. This problem is, however, seemingly caused not by an allergy but by a metabolic problem. The chemicals in question are normally cleared out of the bloodstream very rapidly by a series of enzyme systems which mop them up and inactivate them. Certain poisons, including heavy exposure to the very chemicals themselves, can cause a partial shutdown of these enzyme systems and lead to the chemical sensitivity syndrome. Although avoidance is obviously beneficial, the other mainstay of treatment for this problem is supplementation with the vitamins and minerals which are necessary for the enzyme systems involved. This can take a long time to work, and it may also be necessary to treat other problems such as food allergies or other nutrient deficiencies so as to reduce the total strain on the metabolism. Once again, it is important to distinguish this from M.E. as the treatments are different. However, the two problems commonly coexist in the weakened patient.

The importance of all these problems in M.E. is, first, in establishing the correct diagnosis so that effective treatment can be started. Second, masked and addictive allergies generally constitute a significant part of the M.E. syndrome and treatment of them is necessary for the alleviation of these symptoms. Finally, since allergies constitute a major part of the total strain on the body in M.E., it is necessary to treat them if the patient is going to get well.

Diagnosis

The first clues to the presence of a food allergy can be found in your history. As well as the core symptoms, mentioned earlier, which most people with food allergies experience, many people will have had food allergy problems for years before they developed post-viral syndrome – even going back to childhood in some cases. The sort of problems that should alert you to this include:

Frequent colds and coughs in childhood
Chronic blocked nose or sinus problems
Eating disorders (anorexia, bulimia, fussy eating habits, overeating)
Recurrent headaches
Recurrent abdominal pains
Persistent fatigue
Mood swings
Persistent general ill health

Of course, any of these could occur from causes other than food allergy, but such problems in your past history should alert us to this possibility. The next clue is in the pattern of your eating. People who are allergic and addicted to a particular food tend to eat it frequently. If you write down what you eat in detail for several days, item by item, you may find some surprising patterns emerging. For instance, the majority of us tend to eat wheat – as bread, biscuits, cakes, and so on – several times a day; and we also tend to have milk – in tea and coffee, as butter and cheese and in sauces and desserts – just as often. It should be no wonder, therefore, that these are the two most common allergens in adults. To test yourself, you could cut out wheat or milk, or anything else which crops up frequently in your diet, completely and totally for several days. If you feel better or, more probably, if you feel worse at first and then better, demonstrating withdrawal symptoms, this is a strong pointer to an allergy. Unfortunately, however, if nothing happens, it may just be because another major allergen had not been omitted and therefore the test was useless. It is then best to see an experienced practitioner.

The practitioner who is treating you may well want to formalize this by putting you on to an elimination diet. This means cutting foods out – usually quite a few of them – for at least a couple of weeks to see if there is any change in your condition. If necessary, you may then be asked to reintroduce these foods into your diet one by one to see if there is any reaction. If so, this confirms that you were having problems with the food.

There are a number of tests used to diagnose food allergy. None of them is perfect, but some are certainly better than others. The RAST test is one used in hospital medicine to test for the atopic form of allergy. It is reasonably reliable for this, but is *useless* for any other sort of reaction. If your doctor tells you that a negative RAST test for a particular food means you have no reaction to it, you can rest assured that he is mistaken.

Several tests are used by nutritional physicians and by alternative practitioners for the same purpose. Neutralization, or serial dilution testing, involves putting drops of a particular food under the tongue to see whether you react, or else giving a minute amount by superficial injection. This can also be used for treatment, and having tested and found a positive reaction, the practitioner usually suggests that you have a bottle of the drops to use at home. Our experience, and the scientific research that has been done, shows that this is not very accurate as a form of diagnosis and is a very expensive spiral to get into for treatment. It is, however, quite prompt in producing an improvement in symptoms.

Applied kinesiology, or muscle testing, has achieved great popularity over the past few years. Although in some people's hands it seems to be very successful, we find it difficult to advocate it wholeheartedly. Scientific tests have so far failed to produce any evidence of its efficacy, and it seems clear that it depends very much on the relationship between the practitioner and the patient.

The same criticisms must apply to Vega testing, which relies on the changes of currents through the skin at certain acupuncture points in response to exposure to the suspected food. Also, as a Christian BD remains unsure of what powers are being used by these techniques and is therefore not happy to be involved.

The form of testing of which we both have most experience, because we find it the most useful, is the cytotoxic test. This is based on taking a blood sample and examining it under the microscope to see whether the white blood cells react to a particular food or not. Although it is not totally reliable, it is certainly sufficiently so to be a valuable diagnostic tool for an experienced practitioner. At first sight it is expensive, costing a minimum of around seventy pounds, but it has the advantage that it tests for a range of around sixty or more foods at one time. With all the other methods, except RAST testing, of course, each food has to be tested individually, and the time and cost can mount up to be far greater.

Treatment

There are three approaches to treating food allergy, and we shall consider them in turn.

1. Elimination of the foods causing the reactions
2. Desensitization against the allergies
3. Improvement of general health and nutrition to assist the body in coping.

It is in almost all cases necessary and advisable to do all three of these.

Elimination is the simplest step to take in dealing with an allergy. It is also the most demanding for you, the patient. As well as the likelihood of withdrawal symptoms in the first few days or occasionally weeks, there is the inconvenience of buying and preparing a restricted diet probably radically different from that of the rest of your household.

It can also create new problems of nutritional deficiency, due to the list of nutrient-bearing foods that you may have to give up. For these reasons, the help of a competent practitioner cannot be too strongly recommended.

In general, the results of an elimination diet are, first, that after the withdrawal period the symptoms improve. Second, it may or may not happen that the allergy reduces over a period of a few months.

In the case of M.E. patients, this is unlikely to occur until the other problems involved in this disorder are dealt with. For this reason, it can only be regarded as the first step in dealing with your allergy.

The next step, in the majority of cases, is desensitization. We can leave aside the conventional desensitization practised by GPs and hospitals, as this is only really appropriate for atopic allergies, and in any case it is hardly practised these days due to its unfortunate and dangerous side effects. There are alternative methods, using homoeopathy or kinesiology, for example, which you may be offered. We would have to say that our experience of these is that their success is patchy. In some cases, they have been dramatically successful, but in most cases they have produced little or no benefit at all.

The same criticisms, and some others, can be applied to neutralization therapy. The testing sessions are exhausting for anyone, but particularly so for M.E. sufferers. The result can in some cases be very good, but in the majority it will be only mildly successful. There is also a small risk that it may make you seriously worse. The main problem, we feel, is that the treatment course goes on over months and years and is likely to become increasingly time-consuming, expensive and difficult, and does not lead to an independence but to an increasing dependence on treatment.

The method that we would both wholeheartedly recommend, and which we both use in our practices, is EPD (enzyme potentiated desensitization). This was developed within the conventional medical scientific establishment at St Mary's Hospital about twenty years ago for hayfever and then other atopic allergies. It was later used to treat food allergy. In 1985 BD began to experiment using this treatment on herself and then on many patients, developing the role of this treatment in M.E. It is now being applied to many thousands of patients with a good result.

The treatment is a complex mixture consisting of extremely dilute extracts of most foods, combined with an enzyme (ß glucuronidase) which potentiates, or activates, the immune system's ability to respond to the food dilutions. It is applied either by a very small injection under the skin, or by applying a small plastic 'cup' to a scraped patch of skin, on the undersurface of the forearm. Starting with doses about every two months, most people settle down to treatment every three months or more. After each dose, there tends to be a reaction, which is in effect a withdrawal period, lasting a few days. You should then feel better for several weeks, and the next dose is usually timed to be given just when the effect of the last one is wearing off.

There is a continuous programme of development going on with EPD, and we are now aware of a number of factors that can influence the treatment for better or for worse, all of which are taken into consideration. The drawbacks are that it is fairly expensive (it could cost from two hundred to four hundred pounds a year) and that a number of careful steps as regards diet, drugs and nutritional supplements need to be observed to ensure that it works properly.

On the other hand, it offers long-term, steadily increasing relief from allergy symptoms, and it appears to have a unique beneficial effect on the immune system in general, which can be extremely important in the treatment of M.E. Of course, we could be accused of bias, given that we have gone through the time and expense of setting EPD up in our surgeries, but with about ten years' combined experience of using the method, we are now more than ever convinced of its value.

I said earlier that reactions due to the presence of candida in the gut could be confused with allergies. In fact, the picture is, as usual, more complicated than that. Allergies can drain and exhaust the immune system, leading to increased vulnerability to candida. In its turn, candida can also interfere with the immune system and, as discussed in a subsequent chapter, make the gut itself more porous to food protein, which can then pass into the bloodstream and set off allergic reactions. It is therefore important, in any case of M.E. where these two problems are highly likely to coexist, that the candida should be treated as well as the allergies, otherwise improvement will be hard to achieve.

Similarly, we discussed the interaction of nutrition with the immune system, and it is clear that an immune system which is hampered by poor nutrition will be much less able to recover full health. Moreover, EPD demands a complex response from the body, and to achieve such a response a good level of nutrition is necessary. We would hold back from using EPD when an M.E. sufferer is particularly weak, as the treatment can demand too much from someone whose resources are already depleted, and could precipitate them into a reaction. Before embarking on EPD in such a case, we would try to build up the nutritional status and general health to a level where we felt it could be handled.

Using all of these techniques together, there are very few M.E.

sufferers who cannot be helped significantly. Treatment of the food allergies will not cure the M.E. on its own, but it is an essential component in the overall treatment.

7 Help from nutrition

When Juliet was thirteen she was a healthy young girl, keen on sports and generally liked by everybody. But she developed pains in her abdomen, vague and indefinite at first, which slowly got worse over about three months. She lost her appetite, her weight went down by half a stone and she became more and more unwell. Eventually, she was admitted to hospital and it was decided that an exploratory operation on the abdomen was the only way to establish what was going on. When she was opened up, the surgeon found a congenital abnormality called a Meckel's diverticulum, which is something like an appendix. It had become impacted with food items and inflamed, and had started to infect the tissues around it. Fortunately, the surgeon was able to remove it, and her abdominal pains cleared up. But she was so exhausted by the illness and the operation that her recovery was poor, and she remained listless and weak. She went back to school but was unable to do sports, and her performance in class was always poor. Then she developed a wound infection which, despite several courses of antibiotics, refused to clear up.

Her parents brought her to me, and we ran some tests on her state of nutrition. These showed that she was deficient in a number of vitamins and minerals.

She was started on oral vitamin supplements and we also gave her some injections of vitamins. After the first one of these, she immediately felt better, and after two weeks it was clear that her wound was starting to heal. Within six weeks she was back to normal health and keen to resume full activity. Her surgeon was delighted to see this, as he had been at a loss as to how to help her.

Since then I have had several children of about the same age brought to me with similar problems, but in nearly every case their parents have suspected that the child has M.E. Fortunately for them, they didn't, and vitamin treatment cleared all of them up within a matter of a very few weeks. This is a clear example of the importance of nutrition in circumstances of physical stress on the body, and of the power of nutritional therapy to correct such problems.

Depleting factors

Any form of physical or mental stress places an increased demand on our metabolisms. Our bodies work overtime to deal with the increased workload, or the infection, or simply the large amounts of adrenalin circulating through our systems. The longer the problem continues, the more we use up our reserves of nutrients and become deficient.

The lack of essential nutrients means that our bodies are unable to function properly, and it becomes increasingly hard even to deal with the demands of everyday life.

In no area is this more true than in M.E., because several different systems of our bodies have gone wrong at the same time and each of the component problems can make the other ones worse. So the whole thing can build into a downward spiral of illness and exhaustion.

People with M.E. have chronic and often multiple infections. The effort of attempting to deal with these infections means that your metabolism has to work overtime, and therefore it uses up more vitamins and minerals in order to make the various enzymes work. The more they are used, the more these essential nutrients are likely to be excreted from the body, causing a worsening of the deficiencies. To make things even worse, when certain nutrients are depleted, the body often tries to use alternative mechanisms to do the necessary work, and this can cause depletion of other nutrients as well.

Feeling generally ill because of the infections, you will probably find your appetite is impaired, and it may be difficult to eat a healthy diet adequate in the nutrients needed for normal health, never mind those needed for the increased demands of M.E. Or, even more commonly, you may just be too tired to bother and simply live on junk food and take-aways. One of the areas most hit by this can be the immune system, and particularly the white cells of the body.

The white cells are an essential part of any attempt to deal with an infection or an allergy. They are also heavy consumers of vitamin C. The amount of vitamin C that they need can, in circumstances of infection, go up ten- or even a hundred-fold. This may mean that your requirement for vitamin C goes up far beyond the amount that can be obtained in your diet. With insufficient vitamin C available for the white cells to do their job, the infections may be impossible to eradicate, and will simply continue to make you ill.

Most people with M.E. have hidden allergies, particularly to foods, and these too raise problems in a number of ways. They can interfere with the functioning of the gut, making it more porous to food proteins, which then pass across into the bloodstream and set off further allergic reactions in the already disordered immune system. The gut also becomes quite clearly less efficient at extracting the nutrition from the food that we do eat. Doctors working in the field of nutritional medicine find that patients very often become deficient in particular nutrients when they are allergic to the major sources of those nutrients. For example, if you are allergic to both fish and carrots, then your two major potential sources of vitamin A in the diet are compromised and a deficiency becomes likely.

Allergies also usually lead to addictions. When we identify those foods to which a patient is allergic, we tend to find that the list includes two categories; first, those foods of which the patient says, 'That has always disagreed with me,' or 'I have known that that food upsets me for some time now, and I don't eat it.' The second group is those foods that the patient is eating most of the time and regards as his or her staple diet, and to which, when questioned more closely, the patient usually confesses an addiction. The simple result of an addiction is distortion of the diet; instead of eating a good wide range of foods with a varied nutritional content, the tendency is to eat those foods to which there is an allergy and therefore an addiction. As a result, most of the food entering the stomach is going to set up a reaction, and the absorption of nutrients is still further damaged.

In M.E. there is nearly always a disturbance of the normal organisms of the bowel; this is discussed in detail in Chapters 9 and 10. One of the important roles of the normal, healthy organisms in the bowel is to manufacture vitamins from the food that we eat. Another is to help in the breakdown of proteins and carbohydrates. When these beneficial effects are lost, the absorption of nutrients is threatened and yet another cause of deficiency arises. Besides, having candida or any other abnormal organism in the bowel is an infection which the body attempts, albeit unsuccessfully, to fight, with further nutrients being used up in the process.

The psychological and physical exhaustion of M.E. also means that it can be tremendously hard to eat a healthy diet, even if you know what that diet should be. In addition, the lack of exercise – because exercise makes M.E. sufferers seriously worse – causes the bowel to become sluggish, and this interferes still further with the digestion.

For a number of reasons, then, M.E. sufferers find it extremely hard to eat a diet which will give them sufficient nutrients. The consequent deficiencies make the systems of the body work even less efficiently. The immune system does not work properly, shows even further signs of stress and fails to get rid of the inevitable infections. The food allergies continue and may get worse, creating even further demands on the immune system. The digestive system is unable to manufacture the proteins that it needs to perform its functions because the necessary ingredients are not there. So each problem in M.E. interacts with and compounds another. In many cases, this is made even worse by the presence in the gut of parasites such as amoebae, which interfere even more with the absorption of nutrients. Parasites can also tamper with the immune system to make the bowel a more hospitable environment both for themselves and for infections such as candida. (This is considered more closely in Chapter 11.)

For all these reasons, we now know that a crucial part of the treatment of M.E. is to attempt to get adequate nutrients into the system; but it may require special measures to achieve this.

Fortunately, there are a number of such measures, and we are starting to apply them with success to large numbers of M.E. sufferers. Even larger numbers are attempting to apply nutrition to the problem by themselves. Although it is difficult to do a really good job without expert help, it is certain that many patients do achieve some progress along the road to health. The past few years have been what the Americans call a learning experience for healers and sufferers alike. We now have a reasonable idea of where the problems lie, and of what to do to target them nutritionally. In this chapter we shall try and tell you what is known about these needs, and the measures for dealing with them. To go into the biochemistry of every individual nutrient would require several books, so we shall be concentrating on their importance in M.E.

Replacing the lost nutrients

The first thing to understand about essential nutrients is that they are – all of them – essential. We need adequate supplies of every single nutrient in order for our bodies to function effectively. Some of our biochemical systems use only one vitamin or mineral, some use two, and some use many. So it may be futile to take large quantities of B vitamins, for example, if it is zinc or vitamin C or magnesium that we are lacking. If this is true in health, then it is many times more so in M.E.

But a problem in one area of the biochemistry can cause ripples to spread outwards into all the others. When we are ill, or our bodies are malfunctioning in some way, then not only do our requirements of certain individual nutrients go up dramatically, but a number of other nutrients may become essential. This happens both because we use up our very limited stores of certain nutrients in such circumstances and also because our bodies in normal health manage to manufacture some of these essential chemicals, but in ill health may have difficulty keeping up the pace. The third important point is that although nutritional medicine is all about diet and its effects, nutritional physicians are prepared when it is necessary to use nutrients in very high doses, not to correct a deficiency but as a natural form of medicine. For example, when we use several grams or more a day of vitamin C to combat an infection, we are not trying to correct a deficiency and bring the immune system back to normal; we are trying to stimulate it into increased activity so that it will kill the infection more rapidly.

A final point to consider is that nutrients interact. They interact when they are incorporated into our enzyme systems, to allow our bodies to function properly; but they can also interact negatively, against each other.

This may be in the form of minerals competing for the sites through which they will be absorbed from the intestine, with the result that taking two minerals at once, such as iron and zinc, may impair our absorption of both. It may also be in the form of a balance in our bodies, such as between the levels of zinc and copper, which need to be maintained. If it tips too far either way, symptoms may result. Supplementing the deficient mineral of the pair also tends to push the high-level one out of the system, and both levels have to be brought back to normal. It is because all these aspects have to be considered that expert help is often needed in using nutritional therapy, and indeed the experts themselves often need to use laboratory tests to establish what is happening in a patient's system. Also, anybody working in this area of medicine has to have the humility to realize that they are learning all the time, frequently from their patients.

It can be useful to think of our nutritional status in the rather naive terms of a bank balance. We have certain reserves of nutrients in normal health, and provided we get a constant intake, we can stay in credit. All the factors that we have listed above represent expenditure from the account. Too many of them, going on for too long, can force the account into the red. In this case, a normal, healthy diet, which would have served to keep us in credit when we were well, will now only keep the account level, and prevent it becoming more over-drawn. It will not correct the overdraft.

To correct the overdraft, we need a higher intake. If the stress factors, such as infections and illness, are continuing, then we may need to maintain a higher income of nutrients because our expenditure is still high.

In the treatment of M.E. or post-viral syndrome, this can be particularly difficult, because two of the other modes of therapy which are essential also involve fairly restrictive diets. Allergies to foods have to be treated by avoidance of those foods, and treatment of candida infections of the gut requires restriction of carbohydrates and yeast products. Therefore, it is not always easy to eat a super-nutritious diet. In these circumstances, a dietician who is trained in this area can help (although conventional hospital dieticians are, in my experience, often more hindrance than help because of their lack of training in this area of medicine). Intelligent dietetic advice, usually from nutritional physicians or their staff, can help you to find more foods to eat and more ways of making them palatable. It is, for instance, nearly always possible to find *something* from which to make bread. It may taste strange at first, but it will fulfil a need.

It is also important to approach the diet methodically because one of the keys to good nutrition is variety. If we have a wide range of foods in our diet, we have a much better chance of getting in as many as possible of the nutrients we need.

Although diet is clearly important, not just for its therapeutic effects on our body but also for its influence on morale, it is rarely enough in itself to fulfil the nutritional requirements of post-viral syndrome. Very few patients, in our experience, will be able to get well without taking nutritional supplements. There is now a very wide range of different nutritional supplements available in health food shops, chemists and even supermarkets. Unfortunately, it is a minefield, and finding nutrients that suit you can be a daunting task. There are two major problems. First, price does not always reflect quality or quantity. There are a few well-marketed nutritional supplements which provide, at a relatively high cost, only a fraction of the nutrient doses provided by much cheaper products. You will need to be an obsessive reader of labels to select the best off the shelves. In fact, it makes much more sense to take the advice of your physician. He or she may recommend a specific brand; this has the advantage that the physician knows exactly what you are going to receive, its values and its limitations.

(stress)

The second problem is that all vitamins have to be either extracted or synthesized from something. There is a serious risk that you may be allergic to one or more of the original sources, or to the other chemicals, such as binders, flowing agents, preservatives, and so forth which are put into the tablets.

It is therefore advisable to use products which are allergen free (or to be more precise hypoallergenic). They will cost more, but it will be worth it. Lamberts, the front runner in hypoallergenic vitamin production in this country, have released a new specific M.E. formula containing all the supplements we recommend. You can contact them on 0892-46488.

A further method of nutritional supplementation which we have been using for some time now with, in many cases, quite dramatic effects, is intravenous vitamins. It is now possible to obtain almost every nutrient in injectable form, and our experience shows that not only does it provide the same nutrients as oral supplementation, but without the problems of absorption from a malfunctioning bowel. There are two further advantages. To begin with, it gets the nutrients into your system much more quickly, and therefore gives you a rapid boost. Although this will, by the same token, not last as long as the effects of oral supplementation, it is very definitely worth having if you can find a clinic. Second, it gives you the chance to move forward by a large, distinct step, instead of inch by inch. Besides, there are quite a few patients who find it more or less impossible to get sufficient nutrients orally, but who do respond to high-dose intravenous supplementation. We have both found that some sufferers really need an injection perhaps weekly for some time, until they start to hold their own without it. Similarly, patients who have been doing well on an ordinary oral regime then suffered a setback due to, for example, an acute infection or stress, can very often be put rapidly back on to their feet by a dose of IV nutrients.

Another problem for which injections are particularly useful is a seriously underfunctioning immune system. The use of high-dose intravenous vitamin C can boost this, over a period of a few weeks, in a way that nothing else seems to achieve.

Obviously, you cannot administer injectable nutrients yourself. You will need a physician, and certainly one who is very experienced in nutritional medicine. On the other hand, it may be possible to arrange for some of your injections to be given under the care of your GP. This depends very much on your GP, who is also likely to be forced to use less satisfactory nutrients at lower doses. All the same, it may be worth the effort as an interim measure. Another possibility is to see an expert nutritional physician for specific advice, which your GP may then be happy to administer.

A final benefit of having IV vitamins is that you spend a number of hours sitting around in the clinic with other patients. This may, at first, seem a dubious benefit, but most of my patients assure me that, looking back, some of their most valuable support and useful advice came during those initial IV vitamin C sessions.

Mary is in her sixties and contacted me (BD) when I gave a talk to the Norwegian M.E. Association. Not only was she ill and elderly and living in Norway, but she lived in the north of Norway, further from the capital, Oslo, than we are in London! She had suffered from M.E. for many years. Despite my warnings about her age and infirmity, she decided to come to London for treatment. Obviously, I did not expect her to take the rigorous two-to-three-week course of IV vitamin C when she lived so far away. She was undeterred and took our entire treatment programme. This was only a few months ago, but Mary is already considerably better. I saw her last week and was very surprised but heartened by her comment:

'I am so glad I made the effort to come for the IV vitamin C. It helped enormously. The best part of all was talking to all the other patients and comparing stories and progress and having Karen and Julia there to answer all my questions!'

I hope time proves Mary's investment to be totally worthwhile.

8 Practical nutritional therapy

What follows is a list of those nutrients which we know to be important for recovery for most M.E. or post-viral syndrome sufferers, with some indication of why they should be so. It is not possible to list all those which *might* be important to certain individuals, so I have not attempted to do so. Nor is it possible to be certain that all of these are necessary for every sufferer. From our experience, though, it is clear that this is what most people need.

Water-soluble vitamins

Because these vitamins are all soluble in water, they share certain characteristics. Their turnover is relatively rapid, and they are not stored in the body for long periods. Moreover, they all participate in the biochemical activities that go on in the cytoplasm within cells. As we will see, the fat-soluble vitamins have different roles to play.

Ascorbic acid (vitamin C)

Unlike most animals, humans are unable to manufacture vitamin C for themselves, so they need to obtain it in their diet. Everybody now knows of the proposed value of vitamin C in treating common infections, and this ties in with our knowledge that the function of the white cells in the blood is dependent on vitamin C.

When they are mobilized to fight an infection, white-cell consumption of vitamin C goes up dramatically, and a short-term deficiency can rapidly occur. Supplementation can deal with this. It is also of value in supporting the metabolic mechanisms which detoxify your system and cause the excretion of heavy metals and organic poisons such as pesticides. Furthermore, vitamin C is used in large quantities by the adrenal glands, which manufacture corticosteroids to support the functioning of our systems, particularly in times of stress, as well as adrenalin to give us the short-term boost necessary for any increase in energy output – from the increased blood flow required simply to stand up to that required in a fight for your life. Vitamin C also helps to lower raised levels of cholesterol, and appears to have a protective effect in hardening of the arteries and coronary disease. This may be in part related to its importance in the manufacture of collagen, which makes up the ligaments and fascia which effectively hold our body together.

Factors which deplete us of vitamin C are infections; any other stress or trauma, physical or psychological; smoking; and the use of the oral contraceptive pill. For this and many other reasons we strongly advise M.E. sufferers against smoking or taking the contraceptive pill.

In the area we are considering, the major importance of vitamin C is in supporting the immune function, particularly of the white blood cells and the adrenal gland.

It is possible to take vitamin C tablets or powder by mouth, and it appears that the body will accept as much as it needs and no more. If your intake exceeds your requirements or your bowel's ability to cope, then the vitamin is not absorbed from the bowel and it attracts water into the gut contents leading to loose bowel motions.

This can be used as an indicator of requirements. Experience shows that in normal health, saturation of the absorptive mechanisms may occur at anything from 1/2 g to perhaps 5 g, whereas in times of stress and infection this may go up ten-fold or more. Since taking such enormous quantities over a period of time can be burdensome, it is often only really practical to treat by injection; certainly the high doses not absorbed by the gut can be given intravenously for a powerful boost to the immune system.

Thiamin (vitamin B1)

In studies that have been done on thiamin deficiency, some of the earliest symptoms are irritability and poor psychological handling of stress, together with minor neuropathic symptoms such as alterations in sensation and muscle weakness. As well as its important role in several of the body's enzyme systems, it is now becoming apparent that thiamin has a unique role in the cell membranes of nerves. The active form of the vitamin is a phosphate known as thiamin pyrophosphate or TPP. This appears to occupy sites next to the sodium channels in nerve-cell walls, and to be involved in every nerve impulse that is sent. It is not surprising, then, that a deficiency can affect nerve and muscle functioning, and can contribute to weakness and exhaustion.

A depletion of thiamin occurs when the diet is poor in this vitamin; in alcoholism; and in cases of diarrhoea, when the vitamin is obviously excreted before it can be absorbed. As well as its importance for nerve function, it is clear that thiamin also helps the gut to perform its role properly.

Supplementation can be oral or by injection, and although it may be necessary to take surprisingly high doses, such as 50 or 100 mg a day orally, or perhaps half of this by injection, it is relatively easy to correct a deficiency. I do not see many patients in whom a thiamin deficiency is not corrected rapidly by supplementation. Thiamin is one of the few nutrients which can be dangerous to give by injection as, very rarely, a patient may be allergic to it.

Riboflavin (vitamin B2)

Riboflavin deficiency is associated in experimental animals with high hormone levels which can mimic pregnancy and lead to prolonged infertility, and also with an increased risk of congenital malformations. The mechanism involved is not clear. The most important biochemical role for the vitamin is in an enzyme known as glutathione reductase, which helps to protect us against a variety of toxic chemicals known as free oxidizing radicals. Interestingly, the vitamin is actively concentrated by the brain, leading to higher levels there than elsewhere in the body. These high levels are maintained even in a state of vitamin deficiency elsewhere.

Some of the early changes in vitamin B2 deficiency include alterations of mood and personality; photophobia (dislike of the light); and dermatitis. The classical physical sign is angular cheilosis – a cracking of the skin at the corners of the mouth.

A diet which is low in the major sources of riboflavin, which are meat and dairy products, can lead to a deficiency. Such a diet may well be necessary, of course, for somebody who is food allergic.

Nevertheless, it should be possible to obtain the vitamin from vegetables – asparagus and broccoli are particularly high in riboflavin.

However, the common practice of treating vegetables with sodium bicarbonate to prevent discoloration leads to increased breakdown of the riboflavin which they contain and can contribute to a deficiency. Caffeine also appears to cause an increased loss of the vitamin, and the drug chlorpromazine, or Largactil, as well as other members of the phenothiazine group of drugs can block the metabolism of riboflavin and lead to a deficiency.

Although it is not one of the major problems in post-viral syndrome, riboflavin is clearly important, first, as an ally to supplementation with other nutrients and, second, for its role in protecting against lipid peroxidation – the damage to fats and particularly to cell walls which can occur from toxic chemicals. Anybody with chemical sensitivities, such as reactions to perfumes, household aerosols and chemicals, tobacco, and so forth, should probably take supplements.

Pyridoxine (vitamin B6)

This vitamin is involved in over a hundred different enzymes in the body, and is therefore essential to the normal functioning of many aspects of every single cell. It also works with zinc in many enzymes, and we need it to enable us to get full benefit from zinc. Without B6, vitamin B3 is not metabolized and utilized properly either. Deficiency symptoms include mood swings and fatigue, and it is also very important in premenstrual syndrome.

Depression in women on the contraceptive pill has been successfully treated with vitamin B6 alone (although I would always recommend that other vitamins and minerals are taken alongside it). One other symptom of deficiency is poor circulation and coldness in the extremities, and the disorder known as carpal tunnel syndrome often responds dramatically to vitamin B6 supplements. Many people with low B6 will also have no dream recall.

A deficiency will occur if the diet is low in vitamin B6, but reserves can also be depleted by the oral contraceptive pill, as well as by a syndrome known as pyroluria. In this, a molecule known as kryptopyrole, which combines strongly with both zinc and B6, is excreted in the urine due to a hereditary biochemical disorder. This leads to both

physical and psychological problems, and the only therapy is supplementation with both zinc and vitamin B6. B6 is the most common
B vitamin deficiency in post-viral syndrome. Numerous people have
problems in using pyridoxine and respond better to the active form of
B6 – pyridoxol-5-phosphate.

Niacin (vitamin B3)

This vitamin is essential in the metabolism of fats, carbohydrates and
amino acids, and for these reasons alone its importance is clear.
However, the active metabolite of the vitamin is a major energy
supplier in the body, and if a deficiency occurs, then not only do a
large number of enzyme systems not function properly, but the
sufferer will very possibly experience a lack of energy too. It has also
been implicated in a number of psychological problems, including
schizophrenia, although the evidence is not entirely clear.

It is clear, however, that vitamin B3 is necessary for the effective
absorption of vitamin B12, which can have further repercussions in
terms of our normal functioning. It is also essential for the production
of hydrochloric acid by the stomach, without which the whole of the
digestive system is impaired and the absorption of every nutrient can
be compromised.

Absorption of niacin (which in the same and different biochemical
forms is also known as nicotinic acid, nicotinamide and niacinamide)
is blocked by a high level of the amino acid leucine in the diet. Since
this is found chiefly in the grains corn and millet, people who depend
heavily on these grains – those on a wheat-, oat- and rye-free diet, for
instance – could find themselves with a problem. Alcohol also impairs
our absorption of niacin, as does the anti-tuberculous drug isoniazid.

The important areas to consider in terms of B3 requirements are
energy metabolism, both for the provision of subjective energy and for
the functioning of the whole of our body, and the digestion. The
nicotinic acid/niacin form, but not the nicotinamide/niacinamide
form, has an effect in raising the blood-sugar level for a few hours, and
can be useful when hypoglycaemia is a problem. It can also help in
arthritis by alleviating the pain. Moreover, as well as in the overt
psychoses such as schizophrenia, the vitamin has a beneficial role in
minor anxiety-type problems.

Doses can range from a few hundred milligrams to a few grams daily. For the short-term effects such as pain relief and support of the blood-sugar level, it is necessary to take it in several divided doses daily.

Folic acid

This falls into the B group of vitamins, but has no number attributed to it. It is important in preventing certain types of anaemia, but there can be many problems before an effect on the blood picture is evident. When activated in the system, folic acid has an important role in the metabolism of amino acids.

It has been suggested that there is a distinct syndrome associated with its deficiency, which has the symptoms of gastrointestinal dysfunction such as indigestion, bloating, wind and bowel irregularity (we know that folic acid is necessary for hydrochloric acid production in the stomach), and disturbances of sleep and memory. A number of patients with such a set of symptoms have been reported as responding well to folic acid. Women with post-natal depression often turn out to have a deficiency also, and to respond to supplementation.

Deficiency may occur because of a low level in the diet – the vitamin is present in high quantities in green leafy vegetables and in organ meats. High alcohol intake can also contribute to the problem. Clearly, we should consider supplementing folic acid in cases of depression and disturbances of digestive function. In my clinical experience, a certain number of patients have a very resistant deficiency of folic acid and may need high doses of 10 to 15 mg daily, for a long period. It can also be useful to administer this vitamin by injection.

Vitamin B12

Although a deficiency of this vitamin is known to cause pernicious anaemia, a blood disorder which only responds to injections of vitamin B12, many shrewd GPs have patients on their list who are kept well by regular injections of vitamin B12, even though they never show signs of anaemia.

In fact, there are several reports of psychological and neurological disorders occurring as a result of a lack of B12, well before anaemia develops. The major symptoms are depression and fatigue, and possibly aggressiveness and paranoid ideas. However, it seems that a wide range of symptoms can occur, and no symptom is invariably present in cases of B12-related problems. As well as the psychological disorders, interference with vision and with sensation in the extremities, such as pins and needles and tingling in the arms, is common. B12 is also important for the production of hydrochloric acid in the stomach.

It is well known that vegetarians may become deficient in this vitamin, although some scientists think that because they eat more greens, they get folic acid in large quantities which compensates for this. A deficiency also occurs in people who have a malfunctioning pancreas, or who have had part of their stomach removed. Finally, disorders of the microorganisms of the gut, such as a fungal overgrowth, can certainly interfere with our supply of B12.

It is hard to define a set of problems which will clearly respond to vitamin B12, but it is certain that a substantial minority of patients feel better with regular B12 injections. For a number of reasons, my inclination is not to seek to pin this down, but rather to give all the vitamins anyway. Administration has to be by injection, since B12 requires a fully functioning gut to be properly absorbed. Doses should be of the order of 1 mg to 5 mg every few days or weeks. This is far greater than would be given by a GP.

Biotin

Biotin is usually included with the B group of vitamins. Like nearly all of them, it is a co-factor in enzymes. There is a syndrome associated with an experimentally induced biotin deficiency, which includes depression and anxiety, muscular pain, hypersensitivity to pain and touch, fatigue and drowsiness. This may occur to some degree in conjunction with other deficiencies, but it is extremely rare on its own.

However, we now know that biotin is important for our immune systems, and without it the functioning of our immune T-cells and B-cells (another kind of lymphocyte) is impaired and we do not respond to challenges to the immune system appropriately. For this reason alone, it would be important when dealing with M.E., and especially with problems such as candida. Also, it appears to have a direct effect on the candida organisms, causing them to be less active and virulent. It is therefore recommended as a supplement for post-viral syndrome sufferers.

Dosage would be from 100 to 300 mcg daily, and it obviously has to be taken by mouth.

Pantothenic acid (B5)

When it has been converted into its active form, which is known as coenzyme A, this is one of the most important molecules in the body. It reacts with a wide range of other molecules, and in effect represents one of the major crossroads of our metabolic pathways.

It is essential for the Krebs cycle, which produces energy from carbohydrates; for the urea cycle, which removes potentially toxic nitrogen and ammonia from our systems; and in the metabolism of fats. It is also necessary in large quantities for the functioning of the adrenal glands.

Although a deficiency is rare, requirements can certainly go up. It can be used fruitfully to supplement energy metabolism and also for the support of the adrenal glands, which can become exhausted in circumstances of prolonged mental or physical stress. A suggested dose would be 200 to 500 mgs daily.

Fat-soluble vitamins

These are in some ways different from the water-soluble ones. They tend to have an affinity for cell walls, and their turnover is significantly slower. Two of them, at least – vitamins A and E – are important as antioxidants, protecting us against the damage which can be caused by free radicals.

Vitamin A

It is now clear that vitamin A is extremely important for the functioning of our immune systems. Without it, we are more prone to infections and also to cancer. What is more, it is present in high concentration in the mucous membranes lining our mouths, noses, intestinal tracts, vaginas, and even our eyes. A deficiency can create problems in these areas. A good example of this is the case of measles.

When a child who is deficient in vitamin A contracts measles, the epithelium (covering of his eyes) is less healthy, and he also has a poorly functioning immune system. He is therefore doubly vulnerable and may experience lasting damage to his eyes. Vitamin A is also important for the special senses, and a deficiency can lead to impairment of taste, smell and balance.

Deficiencies of vitamin A are thought to be rare in our society, but common in the Third World. Although this may be true in terms of gross clinical deficiency, it is probable that there are a number of people who have a borderline status for vitamin A. A common problem thought to be a vitamin A deficiency sign is that of rough, cracking heels. If your diet does not include vegetables such as carrots or leafy greens, and you have a high intake of starches, then you can create a problem. Because it is fat-soluble, adequate fat in the diet is also necessary for the absorption of vitamin A. Malabsorption syndromes, where the gut is frankly malfunctioning, can, of course, lead to a deficiency. It is less appreciated that intestinal parasites seem particularly to interfere with the metabolism of the fat-soluble vitamins and can therefore produce a deficiency. Finally, if you have a low thyroid function or are zinc deficient, your utilization of vitamin A, once it is absorbed, will be poor, and supplementation with vitamin A alone will probably be ineffective.

It is well known that vitamin A may be toxic in high doses, and it is the only vitamin for which I have seen cases of toxicity in clinical practice. The two cases I have seen were both in very thin ladies with very low deposits of subcutaneous fat in which the vitamin could be stored, who were taking supplements for a long period of time. Therefore, anybody who is on a very restrictive diet and loses weight should be vigilant about vitamin A supplements.

Except in the above circumstances, it is certainly not harmful, and it is likely to be beneficial to take supplements on a regular basis, of the order of 5,000 to 25,000 international units daily. For dealing with acute problems such as infections, when the immune system needs boosting, a much higher dose over a short period of time – up to 100,000 units daily for a maximum of several weeks – is appropriate.

Vitamin A is not safe in these doses in pregnancy, when the dose should certainly be below 7,000 units daily.

Vitamin E

This nutrient appears to have its major role as an anti-oxidant, mopping up free radicals both in the fluid compartments of the body and in the cell walls. It even has a role in protecting vitamin A from oxidative damage, while vitamin A also acts as an anti-oxidant. This function makes vitamin E important for the healthy operation of the cardiovascular system, including reducing the stickiness of the platelets in the blood. The more they tend to clump together, the greater the risk of thrombosis. The white cells too depend on vitamin E to function. It also appears to be able to make a substantial difference to wound healing, and may delay or postpone the signs of ageing and prevent varicose veins.

Although deficiencies are difficult to demonstrate in the laboratory, and may indeed only occur rarely, it is also true that we can often benefit from a higher intake of vitamin E. In times of physical or psychological stress, we can use it up more rapidly, and M.E. is just such a case.

The vitamin E content of foods, particularly vegetables, declines steadily throughout the winter until the new harvest comes in. Therefore, we are all likely to be more deficient in winter and spring, just as we are in vitamin D and some other nutrients. You may have noticed your skin is dry and chapped in March, but not in August after plenty of fresh food and sunshine.

Doses range from 100 to 1,000 international units daily. People with heart trouble or blood pressure problems must not start on more than 200 units, and should build up slowly.

Essential minerals

We are not going to look here at calcium or phosphorus, which are structural in their importance. Instead, we are examining the trace minerals, which all have major metabolic effects.

Magnesium

Magnesium is a mineral co-factor in a very large number of enzymes within the body. When a nerve or muscle fibre wants to turn off a message or contraction, magnesium is needed. In other words, magnesium is the ultimate biochemical 'relaxer'. It is important for both the aerobic and anaerobic metabolism of glucose, and for this reason alone would be important to post-viral syndrome sufferers as regards their muscular symptoms. Deficiency symptoms include, characteristically, twitchiness and jumpiness of the muscles, and in highly susceptible people even convulsions. Magnesium is also important in the metabolism of amino acids and essential fatty acids, and even of DNA. Not surprisingly, therefore, a deficiency can influence cardiovascular health and cause psychological symptoms and premenstrual syndrome.

It is present in leafy vegetables, and a deficiency is probably not rare, particularly in people on a more modern western diet with a high intake of junk food. Caffeine, sugar and stress all cause us to lose magnesium, as do diuretics taken regularly to encourage fluid loss.

It is definitely indicated in circumstances where the muscular strength is low or there is jumpiness, typically jumping at sudden noises such as the telephone. However, it is thought by some researchers in the field that magnesium has a very special role in M.E. They attribute a large part of the muscular weakness to a shortage of magnesium, which they believe causes the muscles to be unable to relax after contracting, producing a highly inefficient, energy-intensive state of affairs in the muscle. This leads to exhaustion, and also to tearing and damage to the muscle.

The suggested dose will probably be in the range of 400 to 800 mg daily by mouth, although higher doses can be useful at times. Very high doses lead to loose bowel motions as the mineral is flushed out, and therefore it is very difficult to overdose oneself with magnesium. There is an interaction between magnesium and zinc when they compete for sites of absorption from the bowel into the bloodstream. This means that taking them both together may be a waste of time. One of the ways that has been suggested of circumventing this problem is to take magnesium for two or three days and then zinc for two or three days, or – easier to remember – to take magnesium in the morning and zinc at bedtime.

You must also ensure that your magnesium intake is balanced with calcium, or you may push your calcium levels down to such an extent that you get cramps or even, like a few people I (BD) have seen, fractures of bones with little cause after indiscriminate magnesium use. You need to measure red-cell levels of magnesium and free (or ionized) calcium from time to time to ensure the balance remains normal when using high doses of these supplements.

Zinc

Like magnesium, zinc is absorbed into the body and incorporated into many enzymes. These include ones that are essential for growth and the division of cells, including the reproduction of DNA and RNA. Cell repair and wound healing are also dependent on zinc. It is highly important to the healthy functioning of the immune system, and in males the sperm count and testosterone level go down, and impotence may ensue, in cases of zinc deficiency.

Deficiencies of zinc are quite common, and borderline states are almost certainly widespread. This is mainly because many of the foods we eat do not contain as much zinc as they once did, due to agricultural and food-processing techniques. Factors which influence digestion, such as diarrhoea, the presence of intestinal parasites and high alcohol consumption, will also reduce our uptake of zinc; stress, injuries and inflammation of many sorts (particularly burns), will cause us to use up more of it. Pyroluria, mentioned in the section on pyridoxine (vitamin B6), also causes us to lose zinc.

The immediate symptoms of zinc deficiency include immune dysfunction, growth failure, infertility, slow hair growth, cold extremities and reduction in the sense of taste and smell. It also shows up as white spots on the finger nails. In M.E., it is clearly essential that an adequate supply of zinc is taken as the immune system depends on it so much.

Doses would be normally in the range of 30 to 150 mg daily by mouth, and may be needed for two to three years. Zinc is best absorbed when taken last thing at night. It is necessary to keep an eye on copper levels from time to time during zinc supplementation. Overdosing with zinc causes copper deficiency and nausea. A zinc taste test available from Lamberts (see p. 66) as 'Duo-zinc' is a very useful way to test your zinc status. If you can taste the solution strongly, you don't need zinc supplementation as your own zinc levels are normal.

(What a stress!)

Iron

As well as being the kingpin of the haemoglobin molecule, iron is also necessary for myoglobin, which is important in muscle energy metabolism, and for a number of enzymes. A deficiency certainly leads, even before there are signs of anaemia, to a reduction in work capacity, brain function and in energy levels. There will also be an increase of the painful metabolite lactic acid after exercise. Children, particularly males, are vulnerable to an iron deficiency that impairs certain enzymes which break down chemicals like adrenalin. The resulting high levels of adrenalin can lead to irritability and hyperactivity.

Although women lose more iron than men, through menstruation, they are less vulnerable to the effects. Other factors which can increase the loss are pregnancy and the installation of intrauterine contraceptive devices. As a result, it is thought that twenty per cent of women may be deficient at any one time.

Clearly, iron may play a part in some people's post-viral syndrome, although it is not by any means the commonest deficiency we see. One of the notable problems with iron is that doctors typically prescribe doses in the range of 200 mg daily. This is far too much; it interferes with the absorption of zinc and other minerals, and typically leads to black, unpleasant diarrhoea. It is better to take 10 mg daily or 40 mg several times a week for several months. One of the very interesting things I (BD) have noticed in M.E. patients is that many of them have low serum iron levels but normal levels of ferritin. Ferritin is the way the body binds iron to store it. It seems possible that either the body is deliberately keeping the serum or free iron low, perhaps in order to starve out candida, or that there is a problem in freeing bound iron, but we don't yet know.

Copper

Copper is important for the metabolism of iron, and a deficiency may lead to an iron-deficiency anaemia. It is also needed for the manufacture of collagen, and without it we may become more prone to haemorrhages and damage to the capillaries in the skin. The central nervous system neurotransmitters dopamine and noradrenaline are dependent on copper for their manufacture, as is the metabolism of fats.

An excess of zinc or of molybdenum in the diet can lower the copper levels, and it is thought that ascorbic acid may interfere with absorption. However, copper deficiency is very rare, except in some M.E. patients with problems with hepatic mobilization of copper. It is more common to have too much copper, and develop toxicity symptoms as a result. Copper overload is associated with many childhood behaviour problems.

Treatment should, therefore, only be given under medical supervision, and would normally be of the order of 1 to 2 mg daily.

Giving a very low dose of copper whilst giving high-dose zinc supplementation is often beneficial.

Selenium

The major, and possibly the only importance of selenium in the body is in an enzyme called glutathione peroxidase, which has a frontline role in protecting us from free radicals. We know, however, that selenium helps with detoxification of the body, particularly from heavy metals. Whether this is a separate mechanism is unclear.

It has been seriously suggested that the low level of selenium in the soil in Britain means that nearly all of us are deficient, without realizing it. This would imply that our ideas on normal levels are completely mistaken. It is a plausible hypothesis, and I would not prevent anybody from regularly taking selenium supplements at an appropriate dose level, even though they had no obvious deficiency. In cases of chemical sensitivity in particular, and of signs of rapid ageing or degenerative diseases, as well as when mineral analysis shows a low level, supplementation should certainly be taken.

The dose range is of the order of 100 to 200 mcg daily. If you are having trouble getting your magnesium levels up, it may be because your cells are leaking it due to low glutathione peroxidase from a selenium deficiency.

Germanium

Although we do not believe it to be an essential mineral, germanium has in the past couple of years been claimed to have dramatic effects on health. It is reported that it raises the oxygen level throughout the body, thereby enhancing the metabolism; that it protects against free-radical damage; and that it boosts the immune system, both by stimulating the manufacture of interferon and by raising lowered T-cell levels. For these reasons it is useful in M.E. and in fighting candida, particularly because it is in itself fungicidal. It has been used as an analgesic and an anti-cancer agent, as well as for general detoxification of the body. It appears to have a characteristic effect in post-viral syndrome sufferers of increasing their energy level dramatically and sometimes their body weight by a few pounds.

Recent press reports, however, have suggested that one form of germanium, germanium dioxide, has been linked to kidney damage. Until it is established that the form available in the UK, germanium sesquioxide, has no such side effect I (BD) am suggesting to patients that they stop taking germanium altogether. Meanwhile, the British Health Food Trade Association has issued a statement expressing concern about the alarmist nature of the press reports, and stressing that carefully controlled scientific and medical tests of germanium sesquioxide have produced apparently entirely acceptable results.

Amino acids

Tryptophan

This is one amino acid that is thought to have a specific role in M.E. It is known to be important in the brain, as it is converted into the neurotransmitter serotonin, or 5-hydroxytryptamine, which encourages relaxation and sleep. It has been used widely to accelerate the onset of sleep, and to make it less interrupted. It also has mild anti-depressant and analgesic properties. For all of these reasons, it obviously has a genuine role in M.E., and has been used with benefit by a number of patients.

It must be noted that there may be a risk of damage to unborn children from high tryptophan doses, and it is therefore essential to avoid it if you are or may become pregnant.

The dose would be anything up to 3 g, taken in the evening shortly before sleep is intended. It can be taken with carbohydrate but must be two hours away from any protein, to maximize the absorption. Vitamins B3 and B6 and magnesium are also helpful in enhancing the effect, but do not need to be taken at the same time.

Other amino acids

Many other amino acids have crucial roles in body-defence building, and we would need to devote a whole book to their discussion. The supplement I use and find the most helpful is ARG – free aminos from the Allergy Research Group in California.

Essential fatty acids

The level of fat in the diet, and the particular types of fat, have a major importance for many aspects of our health. Fats are not only a source of calories in the body, they are also the major components of the walls of every cell, and are used to manufacture a category of hormones known as prostaglandins, which affect everything that goes on in our bodies. The saturated fats from animals are useless for making prostaglandins and are thought to have a damaging effect on the heart. However, it is now clear that damage can be done by a diet too high in unsaturated fats. This provides too much fat in general and, particularly if fats are not protected by anti-oxidants such as vitamins A, C, E and D, they can be converted into a slightly different chemical form known as transfats. These have a directly opposite effect to essential fats, blocking their metabolism in the body.

High levels of transfats are found in quite a few reputably good sources of polyunsaturates, such as margarines, and any heated unsaturated fats. For this reason we recommend avoidance of margarines, and cooking with a natural saturated fat such as olive oil.

There are two main families of essential fatty acids, Omega 6 and Omega 3. The Omega 3 (fish oil) fats are important in the treatment of many conditions, including heart disease, high blood pressure and arthritis, but do not seem to be crucial in the management of M.E.

The Omega 6 series often seems to have many problems. We commonly find a deficiency of delta 6 de-saturase, an enzyme involved in making the usable forms of this fat from fats in our diet. If this enzyme is not working well, we need to supplement the end-stage fat in the form the body wants it. The best way of obtaining this is from evening primrose oil.

Symptoms of Omega 6 fatty acid deficiency include uncoordination, mood swings, dry hair, dry or greasy skin, waxy ears, hyperactivity in children and depression in adults, increased thirst and a craving for fried or fatty foods.

In post-viral syndrome, it is often appropriate to take specific measures to supplement those fatty acids which are needed most, without overdoing the dietary intake. The commonest method for this would be with supplements of evening primrose oil. In many cases, a dramatic effect on health can be shown, and many therapists (BD included) believe that such essential fatty acid supplements are essential for most M.E. sufferers.

The dose range for evening primrose oil would be 2 to 3 g daily in divided doses.

All of the recommended minerals and vitamins are available in many forms and can be quite complicated to try to get in balance.

In order to simplify the supplement programme, I (BD) have developed a formula specifically for M.E. sufferers which is available from Nature's Best (0892 34143), Lamberts (0892 46488) or the Chambers Clinic (01-823 3700). The supplement is called M.E. formula and comes as a package of the three formulations in three bottles. The yellow capsules are vitamins, the pink are minerals, and the white are vitamin C with calcium and magnesium. It contains all the nutrients recommended and several others as well. There is a vitamin capsule to be taken at each meal, a mineral capsule at each meal, and three capsules of vitamin C with calcium and magnesium to be taken at each meal or other times.

9 Candida – the losing battle

Yeast-related health problems have increasingly become recognized over the last few years. This is largely due to the work done by Dr Orion Truss and Dr Billy Crook, who have been working on this syndrome for many years in the United States.

I (BD) have been treating candida for about five years now and have seen over a thousand patients suffering from various candida-related illnesses. When I first heard about the role of candida infection in humans from Dr Billy Crook, I was fairly sceptical but quite excited about it and hoped that I might find a patient to whom this was relevant and whom I was able to help. I remember Billy saying to me that once you start to treat candida, ninety per cent of your patients will have it. I looked at him rather amusedly and thought that it might be the case for him, but would not be for me; however, I would now say that without doubt candida infection plays a role in the ill health of almost all the patients I see. Although their illness may not be directly related to the candida problem, eliminating the candida from their body and its related consequences has certainly been one of the factors in their recovery.

Candida is a yeast which lives in the gut; probably in God's ideal world none of us were meant to have candida, but in the reality of the twentieth century every person alive is likely to have some candida resident inside them. Most of the bacteria in our bowel are there for a purpose – to help digest food, to provide vitamins and to keep the status quo inside our bowel. These are healthy bacteria, such as *Lactobacillus acidophilus*, which we are supposed to carry around with us. Whether the amount of candida we carry with us is normal or abnormal is a question that, without being able to turn back the clocks and examine our prehistoric ancestors, we cannot answer; but certainly it is normal in this day and age for everyone to have some candida in their bowel and for some people to be carrying it elsewhere in their body as well. By normal, I mean everybody has it, not that it is healthy or ideal.

The problem with candida is keeping it under control. Candida is an organism of low infectivity, but if we provide it with the ideal environment and fail to fight it off, then it is going to set up home in our bodies and cause a large number of problems. As the candida begins to settle in, it multiplies and multiplies and we begin to suffer from the symptoms of an excessive load of yeast. Gradually our body begins to accept the yeast as normal rather than as an outsider, and gives up fighting against it. It is then that we really begin to suffer from yeast-related health problems. We talked, in the chapter on immunity, about how the immune system needs to develop mechanisms for recognizing itself and not fighting itself, but to continue recognizing foreign substances or antigens and fighting these off. The problem with candida is that the body has made the wrong decision in this area and recognizes the yeast as friendly rather than unfriendly.

How does it get out of control?

The healthy population of lactobacilli in our bowel keeps the candida under control by competing with it for space. The main reason for candida getting out of control is antibiotics. As well as killing dangerous germs, antibiotics can also kill off these healthy lactobacilli. Gradually, with each course of antibiotics we take through our lives, candida will get a bigger and bigger hold in our bowels. These days, we also do a number of things which encourage candida to grow. We feed it loads of sugar and refined carbohydrates; many people take the contraceptive pill, which by its hormonal influence encourages the growth of yeast; and some people are given steroids, which also encourage yeast growth and proliferation. Finally, the society we live in, with its high levels of stress and pollution, again encourages our immune system to give up the battle and let the candida win.

How do we know we have it?

Like the diagnosis of M.E., diagnosis of candida problems is based on symptoms. Unfortunately, there are no reliable tests, because if we took a swab from inside anybody's bowel we would find candida. A number of tests are being developed which look either at the growth of candida in the bowel or at the body's immune response to candida. As yet, these are not fully available in this country, although they are becoming available in the States. Their reliability and effectiveness is still very limited.

There is also a test, available in London, looking at the amount of alcohol produced by the body after it is given sugar; although this is a test for alcohol-producing fermentation processes, not specifically a test for *Candida albicans*, it certainly can be quite helpful.

Because of the absence of tests, your GP is likely to be unsure about how to regard a diagnosis of candida. Doctors are not taught much about candida at medical school. They are taught that it causes thrush and vaginitis, and occasionally thrush in babies and very ill people, and that is the end of it. So your GP is very unlikely to be aware of the large number of possible manifestations of chronic yeast-related illness.

We make our diagnosis based on symptoms, and most patients are either clearly suffering from candida or clearly not suffering from candida, and they tend to score either more than eighty per cent or less than twenty per cent of positives on the following list of symptoms. Few people have a half-positive score.

Fatigue
Bloating
Wind
Premenstrual tension
Chronic thrush problems
Chemical sensitivity
Craving sugar, pickles, alcohol, sweet foods
Irritable bowel syndrome
Hiatus hernia or indigestion symptoms
Poor memory
Anxiety
Skin rashes (urticaria, psoriasis)
Headaches
Muscle and joint pains
Uncoordination
Sexual difficulties/lack of libido
Muddleheadedness
Inability to find the right word

These are the commonest symptoms in adults. In children, the spectrum is quite different and the commonest symptoms are behavioural.

If you have the majority of these symptoms, and have had a number of investigations and perhaps some unsatisfactory diagnosis such as irritable bowel syndrome placed on you, or no cause at all found, then it is highly likely that your problems are due to chronic candidiasis.

How does it do it?

Candida causes its effect on the gut and the rest of the body in two ways: part of it is the direct effect of the yeast, and part is due to the toxins and waste products produced by the yeast. If you have a significant amount of yeast fermenting in your gut, it will give you symptoms. The commonest ones from the above list are bloating, wind and indigestion-type pains. Most people have these pains diagnosed by their doctors as being either irritable bowel syndrome or hiatus hernia, whereas in fact they are due to candidiasis. Many a patient has come to me for treatment of post-viral syndrome and failed to mention that they have also been told they have a hiatus hernia and are swallowing bucketfuls of antacids each year. After their first visit and anti-candida treatment, they say they feel a little better, but incidentally their indigestion has completely disappeared.

The candida also produces toxic chemicals by its metabolism. All yeasts are designed to ferment sugars, and in so doing they produce alcohol and a number of other chemicals such as acetaldehyde. This causes the more distant effects, such as those on the brain, nervous system and endocrine system.

You are probably wondering at this stage why, if we all have candida, we don't all have candida problems. Well, it is my belief that most of us have, but to a minor degree. The reason that some people suffer from it quite badly is not because they have caught a nasty dose of candida but because their body is failing to keep it under control.

We talked about this in the chapter on balance, and again in the chapter on the immune system. When the immune system is too occupied elsewhere in coping with stress, pollution, malnutrition and everything else we load on to it to function correctly, it may enter a state of tolerance in relation to candida. Effectively, the body no longer has the resources left to keep the upper hand in its battle with candida.

Annabel was a very bright student, studying economics and politics and working very hard. Gradually she began to suffer from a large number of symptoms and presented herself to the college doctor on numerous occasions with skin rashes, thrush, depression, aches and pains, fatigue and lack of concentration. Each time the problem was treated on an individual basis unrelated to the previous problem, and gradually Annabel's health deteriorated until she was really having trouble coping with her workload.

After reading a magazine article on M.E. she contacted me, thinking that this was probably her problem. She certainly did not have a sudden start to the illness, which is the case for most patients with M.E., but otherwise she closely resembled many of the chronic post-viral patients I have seen. I explained to her how we tried to eliminate the candida from people's systems before beginning to treat them for M.E. as this, I feel, is the most effective place to start.

I put her on an anti-candida diet for several weeks, and then started her on some nystatin powder and a few vitamin and mineral supplements. When she came back four weeks later, there was not a hint of any of her original symptoms. Her problems were obviously due to candida, and she was thrilled to get back into the full swing of life and enjoy herself, do her studies, go to parties and have fun.

Unfortunately, she did need to stay on her diet and to take nystatin for a number of months in order to allow her body the chance to recover completely. But she did, and she is still healthy today.

Jenny's was a very different story. She came along about five years ago for the first time, complaining of chronic thrush and indigestion. She had read about candida and thought this was her problem. We started her on an anti-candida diet and some nystatin powder, and she was better within weeks. She did not keep her follow-up appointment, and when I phoned her she said she was very sorry but she was better and did not feel the need to come back. I tried to explain to her that it was very easy to kill off the candida but much harder to keep it dead. However, I did not convince her.

A year later I noticed her name in my appointment book again. She came back and admitted that her problems had returned. She was a little easier to convince this time, and we started her back on the diet and the nystatin. When she came back three weeks later she was a lot better, but I explained the need to continue with the treatment. I arranged to see her a month later, and again she did not come back. When I phoned it was the same story: she was better, this time she was cured, and she did not need any more treatment. So she thought.

It was eighteen months before I noticed her name in the appointment book again, and we went through the same saga. I needn't go on, but I have seen Jenny on an almost annual basis for five years. She sticks with the treatment for six weeks and then decides it's too hard – she is better, the problem has gone away, and she can't be bothered to keep yeast, sugar and alcohol out of her diet or to take the vitamins. Then the problem comes back.

She is typical of many people who, if they only stayed on the treatment for a few months more, would eventually recover – and, unless they really abused their bodies, they would be very unlikely to suffer from the problem again.

Charlie was only three when I first saw him. He was a sweet little boy from a very happy home with lots of love, care and attention. Since he was about a year old he had had recurrent ear infections, throat infections, colds and a number of behavioural problems. He was also bed-wetting and head-banging. The problem that eventually brought his mother to see me was that he began to suffer from chronic diarrhoea. I thought most of his problems were likely to be due to candida, so we started him on a yeast- and sugar-free diet; his problems cleared up within a matter of weeks on the diet and nystatin.

He is seven now, doing well at school, and is a happy, well-adjusted boy. He still avoids having loads of junk food, but it is not a diet that his friends would notice and he is not restricted in any way, although he pops the odd vitamin pill. I am sure that these small changes in his lifestyle will give him the greatest gift that parents can give to their children – a healthy start in life.

Ann Marie is twenty-seven and is a physical education teacher. She was diagnosed as suffering from MS and referred to me by another holistic physician, who thought that some of her symptoms might be related to chronic candida problems. She started on a nutritional, dietary and anti-candida package, and although it is hard to claim a particular response in a condition where you don't know what the untreated outcome would have been, in the space of four years her condition has not worsened in any way. Every time I see her she says that on the occasions when she does try any yeast or sugar, her legs become weak and she can't walk properly for several days. She is very reluctant to break her diet – for understandable reasons.

If you think you may have a candida-related illness and you are keen to get on top of it, then the next chapter will give you more details on exactly how to win the battle against candida.

10 Winning the candida battle

Beginning to get candida under control is quite easy; keeping it that way can take many years of hard work. The steps to getting your candida under control are as follows:

1. Start by starving it out. This involves an anti-candida diet, which we will go into in more detail later, with the purpose of depriving the candida of its favourite foods and thereby reducing its activity in the gut.

2. The next step is to kill what is there. This is relatively simple although the treatment may take considerable time and effort. The aim is, first, to kill it, and then to keep it dead for long enough for the immune system to learn to recognize it as foreign.

3. The next step is to repopulate the bowel with the normal bacteria or flora which should be there.

4. The final step is to help the immune system to recover, so that the whole person recovers and the body begins to recognize candida as foreign, in order to keep it from coming back.

Anti-candida diet

Candida depends for its existence on sugars and simple carbohydrates. In order to starve out the candida without starving the person as well, one needs to change one's diet and eat very little carbohydrate and no sugars or simple carbohydrates. Sugar can come in direct and indirect forms. The obvious form of sugar is what we may add to food or drink; but the hidden form comes contained in so many sweets, drinks, pastries, cakes, biscuits, sauces and packaged foods. All of these must be cut out one hundred per cent. Many people will find that they go through a period of withdrawal from sugar, if they have been eating a high-sugar diet. This can take two forms. Either they will have an addictive type of withdrawal and crave sugars and sweet foods for several days, perhaps even weeks. Or their blood-sugar control mechanisms will have trouble adapting to the lack of constant available carbohydrate, leading to problems of hypoglycaemia for a similar length of time. The only way to deal with withdrawal successfully is to continue on the diet; your body will eventually adapt to a more healthy way of eating.

Your diet should also be quite low in complex carbohydrates, such as fruits and starch for the first few weeks, then these can be gradually reintroduced in unrefined forms after some initial recovery has occurred.

Your body will also probably need a break from yeast in your diet and your environment in order to recognize that yeasts are foreign and should be reacted to. In a minority of people, on the other hand, the candida problem has caused them to be allergic to yeast, and they should keep yeasts out of their diet in order to avoid allergic reactions. Yeast in your diet does not feed the candida, and that is not why you are cutting it out. The purpose is to allow the immune system a complete break from being constantly bombarded by yeasts and moulds in all forms; to allow it time for re-education.

Yeast can come in the form of bread, alcohol, pickles and mould, particularly in mouldy cheeses. Although some people are extremely sensitive to moulds and will be unable to tolerate any form of fermented food whatsoever, the majority of patients can tolerate cottage cheese. After a month or two they can also tolerate the occasional salad dressing or pickle, provided these do not form a significant part of the diet. Alcohol needs to be excluded for several months, and the first alcohol to be reintroduced should be a spirit, such as gin or vodka, which contains far less yeast than wine, beer and cider, which must be completely excluded for a long time.

Bread contains yeast to make it rise. The alternative is to use a bread which does not require any yeasts, and we will talk about this further on.

Bread needs to be excluded for several months, again to keep the yeasts out, and many people find that they are also unable to tolerate bread again due to uncovering a wheat sensitivity, which is extremely common in this problem. Therefore, the diet consists of no sugar, no simple carbohydrates and no yeast.

What can I eat?

Foods you can eat should be as fresh and wholesome as possible. The philosophy in starting this kind of diet is to try and live as if you were in the country and you had to go and catch or pick your food. If you think of this when buying food (I don't really expect you to catch it) it will help guide you to the types of food you should choose and the kinds you should not. In other words, eat fresh vegetables, fruits, meat, fish and poultry. Fish is fine, for example; but fish fingers are not, because they are highly processed and not in the form in which you would catch them yourself. Because of the high level of simple carbohydrates in fruits, I suggest most people limit these to about one or two pieces a day, and avoid all fruit juices as they contain a large amount of the mould which was on the outside of the fruit before it was pressed.

Exactly which carbohydrates you can eat is a difficult question. In terms of simply controlling candida, you should soon be able to eat all complex carbohydrates, such as whole grains and pulses. However, candida in the bowel causes it to become porous, so a number of substances are able to enter the bloodstream which otherwise would have been prohibited. At the same time, candida releases toxins that interfere with your immune function and can cause an increased propensity to food allergy. The end product of this is that most people with candida problems get food allergies, and the most common foods to react to are the gluten grains. I would say that ninety-five per cent of patients I have treated for M.E. are wheat or gluten sensitive to some degree. The gluten-containing grains are wheat, rye, barley and oats.

A common problem when starting on a candida diet is that because you are excluding yeast and sugar, you may tend to rely on oat and rice cakes as a staple form of carbohydrate. Often you will do well for a couple of months, and then suddenly things will start to deteriorate. This is usually because you have become sensitive to oats or rice. You will need to cut these out for some time. If you are already gluten sensitive, you should keep *all* the gluten grains extremely low in your diet. I would suggest the best regimen for most people, as far as grains go, is to avoid totally the gluten grains and keep as varied a mixture as possible of all the other grains, such as rice, chickpea flour, potato flour, sago flour and buckwheat.

Many people can tolerate milk and milk products such as yoghurt and if you are not allergic to milk, this can certainly be part of your diet. But again, please try not to overdo it. Yoghurt is also useful because, if live, it contains the lactobacillus bacteria similar to those which are necessary for repopulating the bowel.

The one carbohydrate food with which I have yet to see a problem is potato. Almost everybody I have treated over the years has been able to tolerate a diet based largely on potato as the source of carbohydrate. This can be in the form of baked potato, chips, crisps, potato waffles or potato-flour bread.

You still need to keep your diet balanced, and because you are keeping the simple carbohydrates out and the total carbohydrate content relatively low, you are going to become more reliant on fats and proteins as calorie sources. This is obviously not a long-term healthy diet, and after several months, when you are winning the battle against candida, you can gradually reintroduce complex carbohydrates (but no sugars) and reduce your fats.

The recommendations I make to my patients are that for the first week they should be on 80 g of carbohydrates a day; for the next two weeks on about 150 g, and then they can stop counting. You will get fewer reactions to anti-candida medication if you have starved out the candida with a very restricted carbohydrate diet in the first two weeks.

If you really crave something like bread, one product which is helpful in keeping to an anti-candida diet is Versaloaf. This is a bread mix based on potato flour. I mix it with sago flour and gram flour to make a delicious wheat-free, yeast-free loaf. It is available from Foodwatch. Its only drawback is that it obviously contains simple carbohydrates and may cause some people a problem early on in the diet. However, most people could probably cope with this mixture after a couple of months on the diet.

The diet which I still follow – a yeast-free, sugar-free, grain-free diet – is as follows:

For breakfast I have two 2 oz muffins made with the Versaloaf mix, spread with butter and sugar-free jam. I also have a cup of fresh coffee. For lunch I usually have fish or chicken and a large green salad with as many different vegetables as I can think of, often followed by yoghurt or some fruit. For supper I usually have grilled meat, fish or chicken, cooked vegetables or another salad and perhaps a baked potato. This is a diet on which, with variations, most people can live for a considerable length of time without any problem. ?!

Obviously, if you are overweight, you should reduce the fats and the carbohydrates in your diet and avoid snacking between meals; and if you are underweight, then you need to increase your calories perhaps by snacking on potato crisps, putting avocados in your salads and increasing the amount of meat. I would suggest that wherever possible you try and get organic meat as the antibiotics other animals are fed are obviously quite counterproductive to your anti-candida treatment.

+ hormones

I also find avoiding mixing starch and protein in the same meal, as originally recommended in the 1930s by Dr Hay, to be a useful mechanism to strengthen the body's defences further.

Anti-candida drugs

The role of anti-candida drugs is to kill the yeast germs. Most of these drugs are rather powerful and can kill the yeast very quickly. If you have a large volume of yeast in you, killing it off very quickly can make you thoroughly ill. It is quite important, therefore, to diet for the first couple of weeks, and in particular to limit the carbohydrates during this time, to starve out a large proportion of the candida before starting on any of the drugs.

There are several categories of drugs which kill candida. They are:

1. Polyene antibiotics such as nystatin and amphotericin
2. Systemic drugs – Nizoral or ketoconazole
3. The natural retarders, i.e. Capricin and Mycocidin.

Nystatin and amphotericin B

These are related drugs. They were both developed by Squibb in the 1950s and have a long history of use in humans for a variety of problems. There are also good toxicity studies on them. There have been more toxicity studies done on amphotericin B than on nystatin, in particular on high-dose, long-term use in humans. In oral use they appear to be completely safe. Doctors reading this may shudder at the thought of using amphotericin B as it is very toxic when given intravenously. It is important to realize that even on extremely high doses by mouth, the blood levels of amphotericin B remain undetectable even in chronic administration. The toxicity which is worried about in intravenous use is not relevant to people who are taking it orally, as it is not absorbed.

I personally prefer amphotericin B because of the higher number of toxicity studies done on it. It also appears to be more effective and is certainly better tolerated than nystatin. However, it is difficult to come by and is only available in any useful form from France. Amphotericin is available in the UK as Fungilin tablets and lozenges. These are of limited value as the dose is very low, and only in a tablet form. The French form of Fungizone capsules will hopefully be available to M.E. patients by the time this book is published, as I (BD) am arranging to get it direct from Squibb. Because of the difficulty of getting Fungizone in the past, I start the majority of my patients on nystatin powder. The commonest problems with starting an anti-candida drug are underdosing or overdosing. The dose of nystatin/amphotericin is quite critical in order to get the best effect. The medication must be in the form of powder or capsules. Tablets are hard and compressed and do not dissolve until well down into the colon, consequently they have very little effect on any yeast which may be in the upper gut. The typical dose of nystatin that people require is four doses of half a teaspoon each per day. These should be spread out as much as possible and taken between meals, as the drugs can interfere with absorption of nutrients. It is best to build up to this dose gradually, over at least a week. The usual amphotericin dose is three capsules of 250 mg each, twice a day.

Many people experience symptoms of underdosing, especially at the end of the first week. Underdosing symptoms include tiredness, headache, lethargy, depression and crying for no reason. These should not be confused with similar symptoms caused by the M.E. itself, but they are usually quite obvious, and usually occur very early in the treatment. The answer to this problem is to increase the dose. I suggest people increase the daily dose by a quarter of a teaspoon *in total* progressively each day until the symptoms have abated, and they find a dose which suits them.

The other problem, which is far less common but certainly does exist, is overdosing. The most usual time for this is when people are experimenting with finding the right dose and putting up their daily dose. The symptoms are very variable, including anxiety, jitteriness, feeling quite high, being unable to sleep and muscle twitching. All of these symptoms are common in post-viral syndrome itself, but having once experienced this overdosing reaction, you will always recognize it. You don't need to sit around wondering whether or not that little bit of anxiety you just experienced was overdosing or not. Overdosing symptoms are similar to drinking one hundred cups of fresh coffee, or perhaps taking some illicit drug. They are clear-cut, and indicate that you need to reduce your dose.

Taking medication in powder form is quite inconvenient. I suggest you mix up your entire day's dose, which most commonly would be two teaspoons for a day, in a small jar with some water, and carry it around with you for the twenty-four hours, taking a mouthful four times during the day.

Another problem with starting nystatin or amphotericin treatment is that of 'die-off' reactions. Nystatin kills candida by making it burst. If you felt ill with a tummy full of candida, you will probably feel twice as ill with a tummy full of burst candida. It is to avoid this that we use the two-week starve-out diet first, and build the dose of nystatin up quite gradually over the first week.

Often, on holidays or going abroad, it becomes even more difficult to take medication four times a day. In the short term it is reasonable to take your nystatin two or three times a day, but do make very sure you keep the total dose the same. Once you have been on a powder medication for several weeks, you can change to a capsule form. However, encapsulated nystatin does not exist. Many patients have been so put off by the taste and inconvenience of nystatin, that they order amphotericin capsules from France, and as I mentioned earlier, these should now be available here. The capsule dissolves immediately it enters your stomach and so the drug is available from then onwards. Tablets are really of very little use as they don't dissolve until well into your large bowel, or often don't dissolve at all and are just passed out intact at the other end.

These anti-candida medications are not cheap, and unfortunately very few people are able to obtain them on the NHS. This is one of the biggest problems in treating the condition. Your doctor is certainly allowed by most health authorities to prescribe nystatin powder on prescription – if he feels he can personally justify it. This is where the problem comes. You may feel the need for it, but if your doctor is not motivated to learn about this illness then he will probably not feel that he can justify such a prescription to the health authority. Therefore, in order to obtain nystatin – or, for that matter, any of the vitamins and minerals we recommend – you may be left with a relatively large bill.

We are entirely sympathetic to this problem, and are doing our best to try and change things. At this stage, all we can say is that the expense of the treatment is usually worth it, in the sense that most people are able to return to work and begin to earn a sensible and realistic living again – which far outweighs the cost of treatment.

I have been trying for many years to get funding to do a trial on the role of nystatin. I have approached the relevant charities on a yearly basis to no avail, and have recently been discussing the matter with Squibb Pharmaceuticals, who do not seem likely to help. We need to prove scientifically the effect of nystatin and anti-candida treatment in post-viral syndrome, and I hope eventually we will find someone to fund this.

Nizoral/ketoconazole

Nizoral is a very effective drug for killing fungi. It is taken by mouth in a dose of one tablet per day, so it is extremely easy to use. It kills the candida by a type of paralysis, and the yeast is just passed with the stool. This is much gentler on the body than killing off the yeast and releasing its toxins. It may sound like the ideal drug, but unfortunately it is not as safe to use as the nystatin/amphotericin group of drugs. It was used on a very wide scale in the Far East when it was first introduced, and a number of cases of liver damage were associated with it, some quite serious. Because of this risk, it should only be used with regular monitoring of liver function by blood tests. On this basis, it is a reasonably safe drug to use in the short term, but should not be used long-term. I often use it for two weeks at the start of treatment, having tested the patient's liver function beforehand, and then retest at the end of the first and the end of the second week to make sure they are not experiencing any problems with it.

In very ill patients it certainly enables them to begin to use anti-candida drugs without the often unpleasant die-off reactions found with nystatin.

Capricin

Capricin, or caprilic acid, is a coconut-oil derivative which, again, seems to be a very safe way of killing candida. The studies which have been done show it to be as effective, if not more effective, at killing candida than the other drugs mentioned. However, it is not so well tolerated and can cause a number of side effects which seem to increase rather than decrease as the treatment goes on.

The advantage, if you can tolerate Capricin, is that it doesn't require a prescription. If your GP is unable to be of help, and you cannot see a suitable practitioner who would be able to prescribe you nystatin or amphotericin, then Capricin is something you could administer to yourself.

The recommended dose is to build up to between six and nine capsules a day, which should be taken with each meal in an equally divided dose. I don't use a lot of Capricin as I am unsure whether it combines particularly well with EPD. Many people also find that they can only tolerate six capsules a day before they get side effects – usually of churning and discomfort in the stomach, plus nausea.

Mycocidin

One of us (DD) has had experience with an anti-fungal agent known as Mycocidin. In laboratory tests, this turned out to be many times more effective at killing candida than either Capricin or nystatin. It appears to have a unique double action, being both fungicidal and fungistatic. This is to say, it both kills the organisms and prevents them multiplying. As a result, the population numbers of the organisms cannot grow in between doses. The numbers of organisms present therefore decrease with each dose, and the Herxheimer (or 'die-off') effect is diminished. Consequently, the unpleasant side effects of treatment are reduced, and in most cases treatment proceeds more smoothly and with far fewer symptoms. Since there are fewer side effects – and it is also relatively cheap – Mycocidin can be taken for longer, and at a higher dose, than other anti-fungals. At present, it is only available to practitioners, not directly to patients.

Many natural foods also seem to decrease the growth of candida, especially garlic and a rather obscure tea called tahebo tea. Although you may well find these helpful, they are relatively minor factors. In order to get on top of a significant candida problem, you really need to attack it head-on with diet and anti-candida medication.

Repopulation

Having diminished your candida population, you need to repopulate your bowel with the bacteria which are healthy and good and are meant to be living there. This is a fairly difficult process. Although a large number of products on the market claim to contain healthy bugs, most of these would be quite ineffective in starting a yoghurt culture – and extremely ineffective, once they have been attacked by the acid in your stomach, at starting a culture in your bowel.

The aim of the products is to introduce the healthy bacteria, particularly *Lactobacillus acidophilus*, into your large bowel. Obviously, the product is subjected to all your digestive processes before it reaches your bowel, and this is where the problem lies.

The two products which I find quite effective are Klaire Laboratories' Primeplex and Lamberts' Probion, both of which seem to be quite effective in introducing the good organisms to where they are meant to be, at least as far as we can establish clinically. Many people with M.E., candida and food-allergy problems do not produce adequate amounts of acid in their stomach or enzymes from their pancreas. This may be one of the main reasons why they developed a candida problem in the first place, but it does seem to act in their favour in allowing a number of these introduced organisms to survive as far as the large bowel, rather than being digested.

Keeping candida dead

If your body is really to recover, it is crucial that, having killed the candida off, you continue to keep it under control. Don't just follow the steps outlined for a few weeks, then decide that you are better and give up the treatment. It won't work, and you will have to start all over again.

The fourth and final stage of recovery is probably the most difficult and the most important. This is keeping the candida dead, and giving the immune system a chance to recover and to learn to fight off the moulds.

If we are successfully to fight off candida and other fungi within us, we need to educate our immune systems to recognize them as foreign. This involves continuing on an anti-candida regime for many months, and, occasionally, for several years. It also involves changes in our lifestyle and a number of steps designed to stimulate the immune function directly.

To stimulate our immune function, we need to keep on a healthy diet in general with plenty of fresh raw foods; to take a number of nutritional supplements as discussed in the section on immunity and the section on nutrition; and to unload the body in general from all the pressures which are keeping the immune system from functioning properly. These issues are discussed further in the section on immunity and the chapter on balance.

Stimulating the immune system to fight off candida can be done in a number of ways. The provocation neutralization technique is quite effective in reducing symptoms from candida, but I am yet to be convinced that it is really effective in producing a long-term cure.

A number of doctors in America have developed specific incremental desensitizations to mould and candida. These are similar to the old-fashioned mechanisms for treating hayfever, and certainly seem to be very effective. The technique which we both use, and find extremely effective although relatively slow in stimulating immunity to candida, is EPD. We use this also to treat food allergy and generally to stimulate the immune system.

It is important whilst allowing your body a chance to recover from candida that you keep moulds out of your life in general. This not only includes your diet, it also includes your house, your garden, your hobbies and any fungi which are on your body, such as ringworm, tinea, nail diseases or vaginitis. The latter should all be treated directly, and your GP will certainly be able to help you with any of these.

It is also important to keep moulds out of your house, such as on pot plants or in any damp areas in bathrooms, kitchens, cellars, etc. It may even involve keeping the heating on a little higher and keeping a window open or having damp-proofing treatment done to your house. Although this may sound drastic and expensive, it can be crucial to your recovery from this condition. In terms of your household environment, as well as excluding mould, try and keep the chemical load on your body as low as possible. To allow your system the maximum chance of recovery, you should stop using any air fresheners, fabric softeners, or highly perfumed products. Your body is designed to fight all these foreign chemicals, and should concentrate on fighting the battle against candida instead.

People who are suffering solely from a candida problem can also improve their general wellbeing and immune function by regular exercise. However, it is quite crucial here that you establish whether you are suffering simply from a candida problem, in which case exercise is beneficial, or if you are suffering from post-viral syndrome, in which exercise is extremely deleterious to your recovery and your muscle function, and must be avoided at all costs.

Candida treatment is difficult. It is long-term, and you are really fighting a losing battle if you are trying to do it without a sympathetic practitioner who is experienced in treating this condition. If you really want to recover from this problem, please try and find someone to help you through the mire.

Ellen's story

My attitude to life has always been: nobody can die from hard work! I know I abused my body many, many times. I know I did more than my body could take, but every time I bounced back after a little rest.

'A little rest' was what I thought I needed when I went down with what seemed like flu on 16 January 1987. The symptoms were aching muscles and joints, headache, sore eyes, stiff neck, feverishness, swollen glands in my neck and a sore throat. I went to bed with my usual miracle cure: lots of vitamin C and garlic. But it did not work. My doctor prescribed antibiotics, which seemed to help my throat, but I felt dreadful. My stomach was a mess too – I didn't know whether it was irritated by the vitamin C or the antibiotics; I had suffered from chronic diarrhoea for many years, but it seemed worse than ever. The next three weeks I spent flat out in bed. I slept a lot, floating in and out of a dream world and the real world. In between, the colleague who was looking after my job kept ringing. I gave instructions, and all the time I was saying, 'I'll be back in a few days.' I crawled to the bathroom and back to bed. I was beginning to get worried because all the rest did not seem to help at all. I just felt dreadful. My daughter from London, visiting me in Norway, wanted to talk; she needed advice. I seemed incapable of even remembering what she had asked me, let alone giving any sensible answers.

After three weeks in bed I forced myself up. I thought if I got up, perhaps I would feel better. I had a shower, washed my hair and got dressed. But that was my lot for the day – I ended up on the sofa. But at least I was up. I went to see my doctor for the first time since I fell ill. She was a young and understanding doctor, doing a locum for my regular GP, and I had never met her before. She did lots and lots of tests on me, but all she found was a low IgA [see page 42] and a positive ANF [anti-nuclear-factor: when the body's immune system is so out of control that it is making antibodies to the nuclei of its own cells]. I had also suddenly developed a very painful shoulder. She diagnosed fibrositis, but I knew that could not be right. Then I got nasty pains in my chest and was sent for X-rays. Nothing. I was sent to an allergy specialist, who prescribed something for my allergies. But three months later the diarrhoea had not improved as expected. A specialist in rheumatic diseases confirmed that I did not have fibrositis. Fortunately, my doctor never doubted that I was ill and she tried to say some encouraging words when I told her that I thought I was going senile. I had problems getting dressed, and it is a miracle I never had an accident driving the car.

My daughter found an article on M.E. in *Elle* magazine and read it for me. I knew then that I had M.E. My doctor had never heard of it, nor had any of the other doctors I consulted. I was advised to seek specialist help in London.

Dr Belinda Dawes, whose name was mentioned in the article, appealed to my common sense: sorting out imbalances in the immune system, giving supplements of vitamins and minerals, excluding suspected allergens, etc., etc.

About six months after I fell ill, I had my first appointment. I was then working half-time, which was really too much, but I was so worried that I might lose my job if I did not try. Dr Dawes sent me for masses of tests, prescribed megadoses of vitamins and minerals, told me about *candida albicans* (something I had never heard of) and instructed how I should go about the special diet and taking nystatin.

The diet was not that difficult and it certainly made me realize how haphazard I had been about my eating habits. Although I had hunger pangs and I lost weight rapidly (which I needed anyway), I was beginning to feel better. The fog in my head began to lift. I had no problems with the nystatin, except that the taste was nothing but *horrid* and I seemed to have a permanent bitter taste in my mouth – but this helped as a constant reminder to stick to my diet.

I'll never forget a day in October, about four months after I started the treatment, when I managed to rake some leaves in the garden without collapsing with fatigue. It was a wonderful feeling. But there were downfalls too: trying to pump up some balloons with a pump, and three balloons finished me in a heap on the floor. But I felt something was happening in my body, good or bad, I was encouraged. My constant diarrhoea had also improved tremendously. My body felt warmer (my body temperature had been 35.4°C – I thought that the thermometer was faulty). The diet and nystatin had done more to my poor gut than any allergy medicine had ever done. The germanium was then an interesting experience; I felt it boosted just about everything in my body. It gave me more energy, my food allergies seemed better, and it must have had some effect on the candida problem. Perhaps it boosted the effect of the EPD treatment too – I don't know. But I was making real progress, eleven months after the treatment started.

Two months later, I was able to start full-time work again! I rest a lot and I need more sleep than before. Fortunately, my employers seem understanding and have allowed me flexitime. Going up stairs and hills still drains me rapidly, but I feel I can handle it. All the muscle pains have gone – they come back only when I exert myself. The only thing which has not improved much is the mental-blockage I have for numbers.

With my newfound knowledge, I have been able to help a lot of M.E. sufferers here in Norway – not just giving support and handing out information, but also advising about the candida treatment. It has helped the great majority of sufferers.

Oslo, 14 November 1988
Ellen Piro
Founder of the Norwegian M.E. Association

11 Parasites

(DR LEO GALLAND)

Intestinal parasites are a common and unsuspected cause of chronic disease. In most medical schools, parasitology is taught by the department of tropical medicine, which fosters the illusion that parasitic diseases are primarily of concern in the tropics and relatively unusual in the developed world. This conception and the difficulties of diagnosing parasitic infections have led to a serious underdiagnosis of parasitic disease by physicians in this country. Intestinal parasites are a common cause of problems such as diarrhoea, constipation, pain and bloating, and also intestinal malabsorption, food intolerance, chronic fatigue, fever and immunological dysfunction. A number of scientists have speculated that the epidemic of intestinal parasites which spread among the homosexual community prior to the onslaught of the AIDS epidemic materially contributed to this epidemic by initiating immune disturbances.

The commonest parasites encountered in the United States, the United Kingdom and Australia are protozoa (one-celled animals). Two of these are so important that everyone should know something about them: *Giardia lamblia* and *Entamoeba histolytica*.

Giardia has a worldwide distribution and is as common and severe a problem in northern latitudes as in tropical places. Giardia infection occurs from exposure to contaminated food or water. Beaver are the main natural reservoir of giardia. They contaminate streams throughout the United States, so that giardiasis has been known as the 'wilderness disease' or the 'back-packer's disease'. Domestic animals are another reservoir of giardiasis, and veterinarians tend to be more aware of giardia than family physicians are. Children are particularly prone to giardia infections, and giardia is the main cause of 'day care diarrhoea'. Occasional epidemics of giardiasis occur in cities when the water supply becomes contaminated with sewage. Recent epidemics have struck Aspen, Colorado and Pittsfield,

Massachusetts. The usual symptoms of giardiasis are diarrhoea, intestinal bloating and extreme flatulence. In an acute infection nausea, vomiting and fever may occur. Chronic infection may produce constipation, fatigue and weight loss. Because giardia parasitizes the upper part of the small intestine, maldigestion and malabsorption of nutrients may occur. A common complication of giardia infection is lactose intolerance (the inability properly to digest milk sugar).

Most physicians rely on stool analysis to search for intestinal parasites. Because giardia is an upper intestinal parasite, stool examination is a very poor technique for finding it, as the following case report illustrates.

I recently had the experience of treating a family that had suffered from undiagnosed giardiasis for ten years. Their problems began in 1978, when one member, a thirteen-year-old boy, took a school trip to the South of France. Within a day of his returning home, he developed diarrhoea, flatulence and extreme fatigue, and within the next two weeks, the illness spread through the other members of his family – a brother, a sister and both parents.

The family doctor suspected giardiasis. He ordered several stool specimens, but they were all reported as negative. The symptoms abated somewhat but no one in the family regained normal bowel function or their previous level of energy. Eventually they found a specialist in tropical medicine at Columbia University who did several purged stool examinations and confirmed the diagnosis of giardiasis. They were treated with Atabrine, a drug that has been used against protozoan infections for thirty years. There was a fifty per cent improvement in symptoms. After three courses of Atabrine the stool examinations had become negative, but no one in the family felt restored to health. Because the stool was negative, no further treatment was offered.

Over the next ten years, all five members of this family suffered ill health. They stopped consulting physicians and went on with their lives but suffered from chronic fatigue, difficulty performing properly in their various careers, and intermittent vague intestinal discomfort. The most strongly affected was the mother, who finally consulted another physician two years ago. He found evidence of vitamin and mineral malabsorption and recommended that she be re-evaluated for the presence of giardiasis. Purged stool evaluations were still negative, so he referred her to my office.

The technique we use involves obtaining a rectal swab. An applicator is inserted into the rectum and the lining is scraped with the cottontip to obtain mucus. This is then examined under a microscope. To enhance sensitivity and accuracy, we use special stains which are highly specific for giardia and which give off fluorescent light under the proper conditions. Using this technique, which is called immunofluorescent microscopy, we identified the presence of giardiasis in all members of this family and commenced treatment. Within several months they had all been restored to the state of health that none of them had enjoyed for ten years.

I have seen numerous patients diagnosed as suffering from M.E. who, in fact, were suffering from chronic giardiasis and who improved rather dramatically when the giardia infection was cured. Giardia had not been suspected because of the absence of intestinal symptoms. Fever, muscle aches, fatigue and night sweats predominated. I have come to believe that all patients suffering from chronic fatigue should be carefully evaluated for the presence of protozoan infection.

The other commonly overlooked protozoan infection is caused by *Entamoeba histolytica*. This organism also has worldwide distribution but tends to be more common than giardia in the tropics. *Entamoeba histolytica* parasitizes the large intestine and can cause colitis or dysentery. Amoebiasis is becoming increasingly common as travel to tropical countries increases. Of three hundred patients in whom I made the diagnosis of intestinal amoebic infection over a two-year period, all but three had travelled to Mexico, South America, Africa or Asia. The symptoms of chronic amoebic infection may be diarrhoea, constipation, abdominal pain, food intolerance, fatigue and various types of inflammatory or immunological problems.

One of the most dramatic cases that I have treated is that of Joanna, a woman of forty-five whose life had been a living hell for the past six years, following a trip to Africa. While in Africa, she sustained an acute flu-like illness with fever, fatigue and muscle aches. It cleared up. She returned home, and began developing pain and aching all over her body, particularly in the muscles of the shoulders and the legs.

She consulted numerous physicians, including a parasitologist. The standard parasitology work-up revealed no parasites and the

Why M.E.?

various specialists she consulted offered her no specific diagnosis. She became weaker and weaker, and was virtually bedridden for a full year. Finally, she was told that she suffered from the 'fibromyalgia syndrome', and began to experience some relief from injections of Novocaine into a hundred different painful areas (called trigger points) in her muscles every week. With the trigger-point injection therapy and extensive physical therapy, she was out of bed and able to resume many of her activities, but she was never free of pain.

When she consulted me in the summer of 1987, I suspected that she did indeed have an intestinal parasite, acquired during her trip to Africa, which had been missed in her previous evaluation. I ordered the rectal swab examination and we identified the presence of *Entamoeba histolytica* in her intestinal tract. Treatment commenced immediately. For the first five days she was bedridden. All the symptoms she had had when she first became sick returned in full force. After that, she was cured. One month later she was playing singles tennis in ninety-degree weather with no pain at all, a remarkable achievement for someone with six years of fibromyalgia.

Sometimes the treatment of protozoan infection produces a dramatic improvement in allergies. This past winter I treated a schoolteacher from New Jersey who had been ill most of her adult life with severe allergies which had often produced life-threatening reactions. Her throat would swell, so that she was unable to breathe. This condition is called anaphylaxis. The problem had become particularly severe over the past several years, during which time she had made several trips to Mexico. She was infected with both *Giardia lamblia* and *Entamoeba histolytica* but was so afraid of treatment because of her adverse reactions to drugs that I actually administered the first dose of medication in the office while she was hooked up to an intravenous drip. Within five days her allergies began to clear. The chronic swelling of her face disappeared. She was able to discontinue drugs for asthma, and as her breathing improved, her energy level improved. Three weeks after starting treatment, her hypersensitivity to chemicals and irritants was so much better that she was able to teach in a freshly painted classroom with no symptoms at all.

When I first began to diagnose and treat parasites I used the commonly prescribed drugs such as Flagyl. I soon found, using the rectal swab to follow the response to treatment, that my cure rate was scarcely more than fifty per cent. Side effects of the drugs were often very disturbing. The patients described above were all treated herbally and without prescription drugs. The herbal preparation which I have used with the greatest success is *Artemisia annua*, a herb used in China for two thousand years for the treatment of parasites. The active ingredient in artemisia, a substance called quing hsao, has been shown to kill malaria organisms that are resistant to all other known drugs. In acute amoebiasis and giardiasis, drugs such as Flagyl may yield the quickest cure. Chronic infections, however, need to be treated for several weeks or months to produce complete resolution. The prescription drugs are too toxic to be used for that length of time. *Artemisia annua* is not. (There are many different species of artemisia. Some, such as *Artemisia absinthum*, are quite toxic. Others such as *Artemisia vulgaris* (common wormwood) are totally ineffective. Garlic and black walnut extract have also been used in treating intestinal parasites, but their effects are not nearly as consistent as those of *Artemisia annua*.)

I have found the results of antiparasitic treatment so useful for so many patients with chronic disease that I strongly recommend any person suffering from chronic bowel disturbances, fatigue, food 'allergies', inflammatory problems for which the causes are not known, or immunologic dysfunction be evaluated for the presence of intestinal parasites. The combination of the rectal swab for obtaining the specimen and fluorescent microscopy for examining the specimens yields results that are far superior to the standard evaluation.

Unfortunately, physicians who are interested in using these techniques encounter a great deal of resistance from hospital laboratories and most commercial laboratories in having specimens examined properly. US physicians who want to have this testing performed may contact my office for the names of commercial laboratories who offer it. UK physicians can contact Dr Dawes. *Artemisia annua* is now commercially available under the name Par-Qing. It is distributed by The Allergy Research Group of San Leandro, California.

Leo Galland, MD
41 East 60th Street
New York, New York 10022

12   The world we live in

One of the commonest types of question that we, as doctors, are asked socially as well as by our patients, is: 'Why are there so many allergies about? Why is there so much M.E. these days when a few years ago nobody had ever heard of it?' Although there are rarely simple black-and-white answers to questions like these, it does seem that much of the ill health with which we deal is related to the deteriorating quality of the world in which we live. Granted, King Henry I died of a surfeit of lampreys, while some of his peasants starved. There have always been diseases of malnutrition and of overconsumption, but never before have we lived in a world in which we are slowly drowning in our own waste products.

More than twenty years ago William Burroughs drew a metaphor for the general state of mankind from the problem of nuclear waste. That problem is, quite simply, that it neither goes away nor ceases to be radioactive. Therefore, it goes on accumulating and will presumably always do so. Exactly the same now seems to be true of many other pollutants, and these pollutants all add to the burden of cargo on the already sinking ship that is the modern medical patient.

Air

I (DD) can remember passing through London on my way back to boarding school and being unable to see the length of Oxford Street for the smog. Due to a combination of coal fires and industry, much more than to the internal combustion engine, this pollution stung the eyes and nose, gave you a headache and quite soon a cough, and killed thousands every year due to lung damage and consequent infections. The smog has now gone, and London is, by gross standards, a clean city. Certainly compared to the saucer of pollution that sits over Los Angeles or New York, it has 'cleaned up its act'.

But modern pollution is less obvious, more subtle than the old smog. There are far fewer large particles, so the interference with vision is less. But the range of chemicals floating in the air is much greater, and the amount that we know about them is in many cases much less. Twenty years ago, nobody dreamed that we in Britain would be held responsible for killing forests in Germany and Scandinavia with our acid rain. Nor that a seemingly inert, odourless, undetectable propellent gas from aerosol cans would be accused of destroying the ozone layer in Antarctica. But every time we see such a phenomenon identified, the question that a thinking person must ask is: if it does that to trees, what is it doing to us? If we are killing off more and more whole species of animals and plants day by day, what are we doing to ourselves? Are the seals in the North Sea suffering from something with similarities – any similarities, however small, that may sound off alarm bells – to the post-viral syndrome?

Driving through Middlesbrough can be a disturbing experience. It sits in a bowl, like a mini version of Los Angeles, and is completely dominated by the ICI chemical factory. On good days you can see the fumes being pumped out of the chimneys and drifting out over the North Sea. On bad ones it sits there in the bowl on top of the town. As you approach on the A19 the sky gets darker and you will probably turn off the air circulation because of the unpleasant fumes.

Is it any wonder that I have seen a cluster of patients from that area, suffering from severe allergies and metabolic disturbances? Surely they are living in a cloud of poison and can hardly be expected to escape without damage?

Very few places, however, are free from such effects. A whole family came to see me with allergies and deteriorating health. They lived on the outskirts of town in an agricultural area. All their problems started on a sunny day, when the windows were open and people went in and out of the garden. The local farmer chose this day to have his crops sprayed from an aeroplane. Perhaps the pilot misjudged slightly, perhaps the wind was in the wrong direction, or perhaps living on the edge of a field you cannot avoid some spillover. Whatever the case, they experienced a heavy dose of pesticides and were acutely ill, with nausea, vomiting and generally feeling sick, for several days. But then things seemed to settle down and it was not until a month later that they became aware nearly all of them were less healthy than they had been.

For some of the family it has taken more than two years' slow, patient work on their part and ours to pin down the multiple problems in their immune systems and their metabolisms to a point where they can be treated.

A mother and daughter came to see me a few years ago, both with similar complaints. They had been, so far as they were aware, fit and healthy until they moved into a house that was freshly painted. They were immediately particularly aware of the smell from the gloss paint; it made them unwell and gave them headaches which they had great difficulty dispelling. Again, the acute illness appeared to pass, but they gradually became aware of deteriorating health, with a multiplicity of symptoms including nausea and loss of appetite, weakness and fatigue, problems with concentration, memory and vision, and a multiplicity of aches and pains.

We did everything we could for them, including nutritional supplementation, allergen avoidance and desensitization, and gave them advice on lifestyle. The mother improved reasonably well and was soon back to normal health, provided she continued to take certain precautions. The daughter, however, continued to deteriorate, and also showed severe weight loss.

In the end, the only thing that sorted her out was a stay in a total environmental control unit. There she lived on a diet of rare foods free from pollution, and the air she breathed was entirely free of chemicals. Even the fabrics that were worn by staff and patients were carefully selected for their inability to produce toxic vapours, and, of course, were laundered very carefully in a chemical-free fashion. Perfumes, deodorants, and the large majority of soaps and toothpaste were banned. What that spell 'inside' achieved, it would seem, was to give her system a rest from all the many forms of pollution that it was having to handle. This made the difference that enabled her to turn the corner and start to claw her way back towards health. Now, several years later, she is just starting to work again.

Not everybody, thank God, needs such extensive or intensive treatment. It does, though, illustrate the fact that the pollution of the air we breathe, as well as of the food we eat and the water we drink, is a demand that our bodies are forever having to deal with, although they were clearly not designed for it. It can add to, and in some cases represents the bulk of the increasing demands on our systems, that can lead to a 'multi-system collapse' – which is essentially how we see M.E.

Obviously, the most widespread and apparent form of pollution is the exhaust fumes from motor vehicles. Moving indoors is no protection; there are some pollutants that are unique to the indoor environment. The most obvious of these is tobacco smoke, of course. One might say that tobacco smoke can generally be avoided, but there are plenty of other pollutants from which it is less easy to escape. Among the most insidious and widespread of these is formaldehyde. As well as being a major component of cavity-wall insulation it is also part of a number of the adhesives used for carpets and the like. Similar chemicals are released from a host of other sources, such as the bottles under the sink: bleach, detergent, disinfectant, cleansing liquids of one sort or another, polishes, a variety of aerosols, and so on. Dry-cleaning fluids and the 'dressing' applied to new clothes also provides sources of toxic chemicals. There is, too, a whole category of 'personal pollutants' deriving from perfumes, scents, aftershaves and deodorants.

As we would expect, the nervous system is typically the first area to show the effects of such chemicals. The immune system, though – which we have described elsewhere as being both similar to and closely connected with the nervous system – can also show early damage from chemical toxins. These cannot but add to the total burden of stresses on the individual – the cargo boxes on the sinking ship.

Another category of environmental stress factor, albeit natural rather than man-made, is the airborne allergens such as pollen, dust and mould spores. While these do not directly poison you, they can at certain times reach such high levels in the air that they overwhelm your first line of defence against them.

Since their major route into the body is through the respiratory system, the first defence is represented by the mucous secretions, the action of the cilia and the effects of rapid exhalation – in other words, runny noses, sneezing and coughing. If the concentration of airborne allergens is so high that these mechanisms cannot keep them out of the body, then the next line of defence, which is the immune system, is called into play. If you think of the amount of pollen that can be seen in the air sometimes on sunny summer days when the light makes them visible, you will appreciate that every breath of such air contains thousands of allergens. However, without direct sunlight, they are unlikely to be visible at all.

Generally speaking, pollens are an outdoor problem and a summer one. Dust is an indoor problem; it can be a year-round one but is greater in winter. In fact, the major difficulty with dust appears to arise from the minute house-dust mites which live in it, and even from their faeces. This is why the night and first thing in the morning can be the worst times for dust-sensitive patients. The dust mites live in mattresses. One mattress can contain tens of thousands of the little beasts, and they are aroused to activity by the warmth of the human body lying on the mattress. They emerge to feed on pieces of skin debris and other human waste products.

For M.E. sufferers, moulds can be even more of a problem because of the cross-reactions which can occur between one's sensitivity to candida and to other moulds. Fungi are probably the meek who are going to inherit the earth. They include organisms that live on humans such as candida, and tinea (the cause of athlete's foot and ringworm), together with other organisms which are the cause of dandruff. As well as the yeasts used in baking and brewing, there are the organisms that turn blue cheese blue, and that grow on the tangerine you find down the back of the sofa two months after Christmas. Elsewhere in the environment we find large quantities of fungi in the soil, and in the damp patches where rain gets through the roof of the house. There are moulds that live on every living plant, including house plants, as well as on old wood, even on rotting rubber. In other words, the world is full of the beasts. Somebody who, for example, has candida growing in their bowel, eats mushrooms and is exposed to dampness in their house can, not surprisingly, be exposed to more fungi than they can cope with.

The final aspect of the air we breathe that deserves consideration is the ions in it. Anyone who has ever considered buying an ionizer knows that there are negative and positive ions, and they have very different effects. Positive ions are produced by electrical equipment and by many chemical processes. They are present in stale indoor air and, in high concentrations, in oppressive weather and before thunderstorms. They can lead to fatigue, headaches and migraines, worsening of problems such as asthma, and to a general feeling of being unwell.

They can also simply lead to sluggishness of the nervous and immune systems. Negative ions, on the other hand, tend to have the opposite effect, making one feel refreshed and generally better, alleviating headaches and asthma, and gently stimulating the system. They are produced in high quantities by running water, particularly waterfalls, by lightning and thunder, and at the seaside. They are one of the main reasons why you need fresh air inside your buildings, and they can, of course, be manufactured for you by negative ionizers.

Throughout the world there are a number of hot, dry winds – the mistral, the Santa Ana wind, the harmattan – which carry high concentrations of positive ions. Research on their psychological and behavioural effects has shown that about one third of the population are particularly sensitive to the ionic effects. In circumstances of high positive ion concentrations, such people suffer depression and even aggressive tendencies, as well as migraines and general ill health. It is presumed that they are the ones who are largely responsible for summer riots in Detroit or Toxteth. Clearly, though, not all such susceptible people react by throwing stones at police cars. If such a person suffers from M.E., for example, he or she may be made more significantly ill by positive ions. The remedy is simple, although not always easy: reduce the positive ions and increase the negative ions in the air you breathe. Fresh air, running water and ionizers can all be used to this end. Since it seems to be impossible to predict individual susceptibility to ions, I often recommend that an ionizer be obtained, if possible on approval for a couple of weeks, to determine whether it has an effect.

Ionizers also have the effect of depositing dust and other particles in the air on to the surfaces immediately surrounding it. Although this can make your shelf or dresser noticeably less clean, it is having a cleansing affect on the air that you breathe. It is therefore useful in coping with airborne allergens, such as dust and mould spores. Although air filters are available to do the same job, some of them remove particles from the air but replace them with chemicals to which one may very well react. They should be approached with caution. Apart from these machines, there are a few measures that one can use to improve the quality of the indoor environment. Frequent vacuum cleaning, preferably by somebody else when you are not there, and regular ventilation of rooms are important. Dust mites in bedding can be dealt with to some extent by the use of tannic acid on the sheets. This reduces reactions occurring during the night, although it does not always eliminate them completely. I have used this successfully with a number of patients.

Moulds require a degree of dampness, warmth and darkness in which to survive. Measures which can discourage their growth include ensuring the dryness of one's house, and the use of ultraviolet or full-spectrum light actually to kill the beasts. This is discussed later on in this chapter.

Water

Since the human body consists chiefly of water, it is not surprising that it is of major importance to our health. Apart from the obvious problems of dehydration due to lack of water, and fluid retention due to a variety of metabolic problems, the purity of the water that we drink is also crucial. Sadly, it is now acknowledged by scientists that there is no completely pure water available in England any more. Ever since the Industrial Revolution we have been systematically polluting our water supplies. When farmers spray chemicals on to their crops, these are washed by the rain into the soil, and thus into rivers and down into the underground aquifers. It has always been the case that water from deep artesian sources has been filtered through hundreds of feet of rock, thereby having all the impurities removed. Nowadays, however, the level of pollution is such that this rock filter is no longer adequate for removing all the chemicals. As well as agricultural by-products, the waste products of a variety of industries have been seeping into our water for decades.

Even the level of radioactivity is rising, as a result of nuclear testing and the general use of radioactive products, as well as of disasters such as Chernobyl.

The principal aim of purification by water authorities has always been to remove or kill microorganisms that could cause diseases such as typhoid. Compared to chemical pollution, this has been achieved relatively effectively. But the cost of this process is a level of chlorine in the water supply which can itself cause problems for susceptible people. Chlorine is potentially a toxic chemical in its own right, and although the levels are sufficiently low that acute problems are rare, all of us are vulnerable to chronic effects as it adds to the total pollutant load that we have to handle. Moreover, people with meta-bolic problems, particularly with the sort of multi-system collapse with which we are dealing in this book, may have more significant problems with chlorine.

As a result, it is advisable for most of us to take steps to ensure the purity of our own personal water supplies. There are really only two ways that this can be done. The first is to buy bottled mineral water, which comes from deep sources of very pure water. While some people have found it advisable or necessary to use mineral water for all their intake, this is expensive and, for most of us, unnecessary. There are water filters on the market which can either sit on a work surface or be plumbed into the water supply.

As a simple demonstration of the value of a water filter, you can try the following test. Using an ordinary worktop water filter, pour a glass of filtered water and put it beside a glass of tap water. Taste the filtered water first, noting appearance, the degree of oiliness and the taste on the tongue. Then taste the tap water. If the difference is not striking, then you have either a seriously damaged sense of taste or a water supply which the rest of us can envy.

Food

The quality of the food that we eat has also deteriorated over recent years, in two distinct ways: the nutrient content has gone down, and the additive content has gone up.

Farming is big business, and it has always required commercial as well as ecological or humanitarian decisions from farmers and farm managers. Nowadays, much of farming is conducted on a massive scale by large conglomerates, and the decisions are much more likely to be strictly commercial in basis. The nourishment value of food therefore takes a low precedence in comparison to the rapid-growing properties or the presentable appearance of a crop.

There are certain minerals – selenium, for example – which are essential to man but not to plants. There are other nutrients which we require more of than we can easily get from modern food. Moreover, once a crop is removed from the ground or from the branch, the vitamin content starts to decline.

Some vitamins decline much faster than others, of course, but decline they all do. A few days of transport and storage may be sufficient to wipe out the bulk of the vitamin C in an orange, for instance. Some other nutrients, such as vitamin E, decline only over a period of months; but then grains are often stored from harvesting time throughout the winter, and by early spring the levels of vitamin E may be seriously depleted.

Food processing also removes nutrients, either deliberately or as a side effect. It may be deliberate in a case such as that of zinc, which is known to encourage the growth of microorganisms on food. Since these microorganisms are largely responsible for the rotting of food, removal of zinc and certain other components increases its shelf life.

An example of unintentional removal of nutrients is the milling of flour. The main purpose of this is to make grains easier to process into flour and bread. This is done by separating the starch from the fibre and the germ. The germ is the actual growing seed, while the starch is merely the food store that nature provides it with. The germ also contains most of the vitamins, minerals and protein. Although government regulations require that certain amounts of vitamins are put back into flour, it can only be a poor substitute for real nutrients.

The final stage in the journey from field to table, of course, is cooking. The boiling or frying of food always removes considerable quantities of nutrients from it. There are less damaging techniques, such as steaming and stir frying, but the most nutritious food is always going to be raw food.

As well as nutrients being removed from food, an increasing number of chemicals are added to it. It is now said that an iceberg lettuce may be sprayed at least fourteen times while it is growing. Other crops are no better off. After harvesting, vegetables and fruit are likely to be subjected to other sprays, including sulphites and sulphates, which are designed to retard deterioration. Unfortunately, they break down B vitamins in the process.

Food that is processed in any way – in other words, food that arrives in the kitchen in a different form from that in which it left the farm – is likely to have had chemicals added. These are used to improve the texture, taste, or appearance of food, as well as to increase its shelf life. The United Kingdom uses 200,000 tons of such additives every year, as well as 26,000 tons of pesticides. Very few of these have any benefit for the consumer. They enable food producers to sell us food which is attractive, has a longer shelf life, and makes a greater profit for them. Some of them, indeed, are harmful. Some have been associated with diseases such as migraine, skin rashes and asthma, and others are known to be carcinogenic. Moreover, it is possible to become allergic to a large number of them. The most obvious example is hyperactivity in children caused by food additives.

The question of what to do about this deterioration in our food has only a few answers. Clearly, it is better for our health to eat better, and we should be making our opinions felt in public, although this is something at which the British are notoriously bad. For the individual, however, this is liable to be too long and slow a process. We need to obtain better food now, particularly if we suffer from an illness such as M.E., to which poor nutrition can contribute, as well as the added burden of chemicals in our food which can poison our body.

The most obvious way to do this is to eat organic food when possible. This is grown without the spraying or other addition of chemicals, and in soils which have preserved the mineral content over the years. Organic food does tend to be somewhat more expensive than 'ordinary' food, but this is to some extent a problem of scale. When more organic food is produced, it will become cheaper. Besides, it is often the case that non-organic food has a higher water content, due to added hormones. As a result, although a pound of organic carrots, for instance, costs more, the nutrient content is considerably higher.

Light

Our bodies have been designed, through millions of years of evolution, for an environment which contains certain levels of nutrients, water, oxygen and other components in the air that we breathe, and light. There is a great deal of evidence, accumulated over the past hundred years, that light is an essential nutrient in exactly the same way as vitamins or minerals are. Unfortunately, ever since the Industrial Revolution, we have been moving indoors and away from the light. As a result, more and more of us suffer from a variety of light-deficiency syndromes.

Over the last couple of years, there has been a degree of publicity given to a disease called seasonal affective disorder. This is a form of depression, but with some physical aspects as well as psychological ones, associated with low levels of light, and it therefore occurs in winter. It can be treated by boosting the levels of light to which a sufferer is exposed, either sunlight or artificial light, but it also requires the right quality of light.

Simply from talking to patients, though, it is apparent that there are now many people who suffer also from a seasonal physical disorder, in which they become physically ill rather than depressed in the winter months.

It is clear that there are more general effects of light which influence every one of us. These include an influence on hormones, for which the mechanism is clear. Light hitting the eye sets off a nervous signal which triggers the pineal gland. This in turn influences the pituitary gland, which is the regulator of all our hormones. Light can therefore be used to stimulate the thyroid, the adrenals, the sexual glands, and thereby the whole of our bodies.

Light also stimulates our cardiovascular systems, increasing the strength of contraction of the heart and thus the blood flow throughout the whole system, as well as reducing blood pressure. Consequently, not only is more blood supplied to the muscles, enabling a greater energy output from them, but there is increased blood flow through the brain, with obvious benefits to our mental functioning, and through the kidneys, increasing our ability to detoxify the system.

Sunlight hitting the skin also triggers off release of hormonal chemicals which boost the immune system, raising the level of T-cells in the blood and their activity rates. This increases our resistance to infection and our ability to cope with a wide range of diseases – including post-viral syndrome. At the same time, sunlight hitting the skin converts certain oils into forms which have antiseptic properties, and this reduces the entry of infections into the body. Since the organisms which cause infections are much more susceptible to damage by sunlight and other radiation than humans are, the level of lighting clearly influences infections even before the bugs get near to our bodies. Naturally, this has a lot to do with the high rate of infection in children and old people in particular during the winter months.

We have always known that sunlight hitting the skin stimulates the manufacture of vitamin D, which is important for our calcium metabolism and thus for the strength of our bones. It is now also clear that vitamin D has an effect through calcium metabolism on the health of our cardiovascular systems, preventing hardening of the arteries, for example. Vitamin D is a hormone in its own right and it has a direct effect on the immune system, regulating the levels of T-cells in the blood, and a specific effect on cancerous cells. In the laboratory, vitamin D has been shown to be able actually to convert human leukaemia cells back into normal cells.

Another important effect of light is on the reproductive system. We know that sunlight and the workings of the pineal are important for the start and regulation of the menstrual cycle in women, as well as boosting levels of both male and female sex hormones.

Finally, as far as M.E. sufferers are concerned, it should be obvious that we all tend to feel more relaxed, happy and healthy after a period in the sun. This may be the biggest reason why holidays are important. It may also explain why winter holidays are a good idea, since skiing invariably happens in mountainous areas, at high altitudes, where the UV intensity is much higher than at sea level.

In our modern world, it is now possible to work the whole day indoors and to travel to and from work in enclosed cars, buses and trains. As a result, our exposure to sunlight may only occur during a few minutes in the morning and evening, when sunlight is at a lower level than in the middle of the day. Windows filter out a significant part of daylight, and indoor lighting in offices, schools and other places of work is always at a much lower level than the daylight outside. Besides, artificial lights provide only a part of the full spectrum of sunlight.

Sunlight reaching the earth's surface includes the whole range of visible light, but this is only three-quarters of the total. There is also another twenty-five per cent of ultraviolet, which our eyes cannot see. Birds, fish and insects can all see ultraviolet light, and they therefore have four primary colours in their vision rather than three. Nevertheless, UV adds a different quality to what we see, giving it sparkle and substance. It also has important health benefits. Most of the effects that I have listed above are dependent on UV and receiving the entire spectrum of light in the correct proportions. You might say that we need a balanced diet of light, just as we need a balance between the protein, calories, vitamins and other components in our food.

Unfortunately, glass in windows, windscreens and even spectacles – and the same goes for plastics nowadays – filters out the UV and much of the blue, leaving us with the green, yellow and red areas of the spectrum. Not only SAD victims suffer the ill effects of this; we all do. Our experience with M.E. sufferers is not extensive, but it seems to be the case that nearly all of them will benefit to some extent from better light, or even light therapy, and about forty per cent of them will benefit a great deal.

Clearly, you can help yourself by going on holiday to sunny places when possible, and even by simply stepping outdoors in the middle of the day when there is any sunlight about. This even applies in winter, although the time when there is enough light around to do any good is very short, no more than a couple of hours, and, of course, rainy or very cloudy days reduce the available light considerably.

The other measure that can be used is full-spectrum lighting. This is a form of artificial light which produces, as nearly as possible, the same distribution of wavelengths as sunlight. Both BD's clinic in Chelsea and DD's clinic in York have full-spectrum lighting. We have also started using much higher intensities of light in a form of light therapy. Patients are exposed for between half an hour and an hour to a unit similar to a sunbed, but without the tanning properties, which provides the whole range of sunlight rather than just a narrow band. Some of the effects on fatigue, tension, blood pressure, stiff and aching muscles and joints and so forth are quite striking.

Perhaps most important of all, though, is a change in attitude. There has been so much publicity recently about the supposed association between sunlight and skin cancer that we are in danger of becoming troglodytes, shielding ourselves from the sun at every opportunity.

There is no doubt that this will be seriously damaging to our health; it is already happening. Unless we come to accept that sunlight is not only good for us, it is essential, we shall continue to damage ourselves and to miss out on a major factor which can make us healthier.

Dr Downing's book on this subject, *Day Light Robbery: The Importance of Sunlight to Health*, was published by Arrow Books in 1988.

13 Partly in the mind

Personality type

Eight times out of ten, people who suffer from post-viral syndrome show certain similarities in personality. I do not for a moment mean that I think post-viral syndrome is an illness of personality, nor do I think that it is a psychological illness, but just as many studies have shown that people who suffer from heart disease or from cancer often have a particular personality type, so, I feel, do post-viral syndrome sufferers.

Typical sufferers are often high achievers who constantly set themselves goals which they can't quite reach, and keep themselves emotionally busy achieving these. They may be physically fit and active, but this is not usually the case. They are frequently characterized by the sort of traits that their friends might describe as stubbornness, pigheadedness or obstinacy, and by an inability to give in under pressure. They want to reach their goal, and very little seems to get in their way.

However, they also tend to be swayed easily by the opinions of others, so although they may seem obstinate and difficult on the surface, underneath they will be striving quite hard to gain recognition and approval.

A lot of the disorder could stem from a deep-seated lack of self-acceptance. They feel uncomfortable about being kind to themselves. When they are suffering from an illness such as flu or a cold, they tend to go on pushing rather than give in and go to bed. This is where the personality type and the illness come together.

Very often the circumstances in which they find themselves before contracting M.E. are relatively unacceptable, but they can't see a better alternative. Perhaps they don't feel particularly wanted,

appreciated or accepted for who and what they are, yet there is
nothing seriously negative to make them search for something better.
A person with high self-esteem would probably respond in this
situation by moving away from it, whereas others might feel it their
lot in life to tolerate the situation. Constant year-after-year dis-
satisfaction gnaws away at the immune system, and makes people
vulnerable to chronic illnesses such as M.E.

Poor dietary patterns can result in nutritional deficiencies. Potential M.E. sufferers, striving hard for recognition and achievement,
working long hours, and having little time to cook, may not feel
particularly good about themselves or their body and therefore may
be quite happy having a pizza or hamburger for dinner several nights
a week. Obviously, this will deplete the body of its natural stores of
vitamins and minerals, which in current times are spread pretty thin
on the ground anyway. Once again, this helps to deplete the body's
immune function.

To make all of this worse, if they begin to perceive the position they
are in, they are likely, because of their achievement-orientated personality, to respond by joining a health club or a gym. Rather than
being generally nice to themselves and cleaning their diet up, for
instance, they will take on a high-pressure, increasingly difficult
exercise schedule to 'improve' their body.

This, combined with all the other factors, is likely to be the last
straw that breaks the camel's back. Many times I have seen people
who fit into all the previous personality and lifestyle characteristics
join a gym, take up jogging or start to swim regularly – and only then
crash and become ill.

Illness behaviour

I've said quite a lot about the typical personality which suffers from
post-viral syndrome. Such people, when they get ill, may have one of
several characteristic reactions. The commonest is to ignore the
illness completely. This is ideal for getting the post-viral syndrome
established; if they had gone to bed and behaved in what might
appear to be a childish manner, the illness probably wouldn't have
got a hold to start with.

Ignoring that there is anything wrong, carrying on working, and
even carrying on exercising, is quite a common response. Probably

even more common are the sufferers who respond by having only two or three days in bed, when they would obviously be better off with a week. They feel guilty at having let down their colleagues, or worry what the boss might be thinking, so they return to work not only far sooner than they should, but with a burden of guilt for having let the side down, and with a need to catch up on what they missed during the few days they were off. This, too, is the sort of behaviour that encourages post-viral syndrome to become established.

Very often, when these people realize they are ill and have lost a degree of control over their lives, everything begins to crumble. They are no longer getting the results they need to achieve, so they are not getting the approval and recognition that they crave from others and this makes the downward spiral even worse.

Changes needed

In order to recover from post-viral syndrome, an enormous amount of change has to be instituted. Most of this change is in the areas of diet, nutrition and lifestyle – learning to adapt to the illness. However, there are some crucial adjustments that may need to be made to your entire attitude and outlook on life. These are discussed in further detail in chapter 12.

Not only do you need to change your eating patterns, lifestyle and behaviour, you also need to change the thinking behind the behaviour. People suffering from post-viral syndrome commonly seek the approval of others, and when they lose this they lose their definition of themselves. The first step in therapy is therefore working out exactly who you are.

The next major step is learning to like yourself. This can be an enormous leap if you have spent twenty or thirty years in a personality struggle based on not liking yourself and in a constant search for the approval of others.

In order to recover, these problems need to be addressed. I (BD) refer a number of patients to traditional long-term psychotherapy. I also refer a number to much shorter courses of psychotherapy, which are probably more effective in this situation. The sort of person who suffers from post-viral syndrome is usually intelligent and responds better to a more structured therapy than to the lengthy wanderings of classical analysis.

A form of therapy which I have found helpful to some patients is rebirthing. Although this sounds bizarre, the name is fairly inappropriate; the treatment involves discussions with a therapist, and then a course of relaxation and deep breathing after the discussion, while a number of these ideas are churned around in your mind, and then another period of discussion. I feel therapies are more effective where the therapist takes an active role in helping to uncover particular behaviour patterns that seem to be encouraging the illness to continue, rather than sitting mute for several years, listening.

The other form of therapy which I think is also very useful is Inner Healing. This is the name for Christian prayer ministry which is conducted by trained counsellors, not for a specific virus or other physical problem, but to deal with the emotional hurts and past problems which may be helping to create a situation where the illness can take hold, and to ask God to intervene and heal these hurts and cure the illness.

Depression

Depression is surprisingly uncommon in post-viral syndrome. When successful, ambitious, intelligent people are struck down in the prime of life, and become unable to do much more than bath and dress themselves, you could expect them to become depressed.

I'm not sure why people with post-viral syndrome are so rarely depressed. At a deep level, I think many patients have a fairly resigned attitude to the illness. Depression as a primary illness, rather than a response to the post-viral syndrome, is extremely uncommon in this condition, and I would postulate that the person with post-viral syndrome does not become depressed, he or she gets post-viral syndrome instead, as they have a different mechanism for somatizing their stress. Nevertheless, a number of people find that antidepressants help a little – although I haven't seen any very dramatic response to them. The one I use most commonly is Prothiaden and the dose is 75 milligrams each night.

Many GPs think patients with post-viral syndrome are simply depressed, and refer them to a psychiatrist. Fortunately, more and more psychiatrists are coming to recognize that post-viral syndrome exists, but we have heard some hair-raising stories from M.E. patients referred to psychiatrists who didn't recognize the condition.

At the request of family and friends who felt they were suffering from post-viral syndrome, I have been to see (with the permission of their psychiatrists) a number of people on their first few visits as in-patients in psychiatric hospitals. Only if the psychiatrist agrees have I been able to institute any treatment for their post-viral syndrome, but I think I can say that all the patients I have seen in this situation have recovered.

Amanda's story

In February 1986 I went skiing in France. I arrived feeling tired after a busy few months at work, but I was looking forward to a week's skiing in the Alps. After dinner on the first night, I was violently sick, and the following morning I woke up with an acute sore throat and a heavy cold. It was a miserable holiday and I came back to England to spend another week in bed. Having had several bouts of glandular-fever-type illnesses, my symptoms (except for the sickness and continual feeling of nausea) were depressingly familiar.

However, I seemed to recover, and it was not until the following May that I began to feel nauseous and feverish again. My GP clearly thought that I was a stressed and neurotic female and sent me off for tests for an ulcer – I thought this most unlikely as I had no pain and my symptoms could occur at any time, not just when I was under stress. I was losing weight and I looked terrible, I had no energy and was permanently exhausted.

I was still working and hoping the problem would go away when I collapsed in mid-October with what I later found out was an anxiety attack. At the time I thought I must be having a breakdown – I had never ever experienced anything like it before and I was terrified. My mother came to stay with me and together we went back to my GP. He recommended that I should see a psychiatrist, and if I could go privately, I could see him that afternoon. My mother and I agreed, although by this time I was feeling so shell-shocked that I wasn't really aware of anything except that all I wanted to do was abdicate all responsibility for myself.

The psychiatrist admitted me to a private psychiatric clinic the following day. Needless to say, I felt horrified and embarrassed at the thought of having a 'psychiatric' problem, but I immediately felt more secure in the clinic than at home, and I slowly began to calm down.

The psychiatrist very quickly told me that in his view I was not suffering from any mental illness or emotional trauma and that my illness must be organic. He arranged for me to have numerous blood tests and he came back later that week to tell me that I appeared to have a chronic infection. It was an enormous relief to know that my illness really was genuine and that it had a name (even if there was no treatment or cure for it). I had always known that there was something organically wrong with me and that I wasn't malingering or suffering from emotional stress.

Very fortunately for me, my psychiatrist had recently seen a similar case to mine and he was able to put me in touch with Dr Belinda Dawes, who diagnosed me at once as having M.E. I stayed in the clinic for several weeks just resting while I started Dr Dawes' treatment.

Having my M.E. diagnosed in a psychiatric clinic certainly wasn't ideal, but I am immensely grateful to my psychiatrist for his help and understanding in recognizing that I had a real illness, something that my NHS GP had singularly failed to do.

Inevitably with M.E., it has been a long haul, but I am now, since Dr Dawes' treatment, feeling far stronger and at times really well. I still go up and down, and I still need a lot of rest and sleep, but I am sure that I will eventually make a full recovery.

Prayer/support

There is a great need in people with post-viral syndrome to talk to other sufferers. This is similar to the situation in Alcoholics Anonymous and Weight Watchers; initially, people are reticent to meet others with the condition, as their response to the illness is very much in keeping with their personality type, which is to ignore the illness or to make as little allowance for it as possible. Therefore, the majority of people do not wish to become part of any organized structure associated with their illness.

I can entirely understand this philosophy, but I think that people who make the jump and join with other sufferers on a regular basis do gain a lot by shared experiences, and by the support that this can generate.

The practice that I (BD) run, treating post-viral syndrome, is a Christian practice, and I hope that we provide a service in terms of support. As well as three trained nurses, we have a trained Christian counsellor on the staff who is available to take people on for longer sessions of counselling or ministry – which we encourage all patients to embark upon, either with us, or with a number of other therapists to whom I recommend people.

We also run a support group which meets one Sunday of the month for people to get together and discuss their problems, feelings and treatments with each other.

Chat lines

The M.E. Association and the M.E. Action Campaign both have telephone lines which you can ring at almost any time to discuss your problems or your illness with a sympathetic counsellor or fellow sufferer. The number of the M.E. Association line is: 0375 642466. The number of the M.E. Action Campaign is not yet finalized but will be notified to those on their mailing list as soon as it is.

These two groups also run local support groups throughout the country, and many people find a lot of benefit from joining them. You can find out more about them by writing to the M.E. Association at PO Box 8, Stanford le Hope, Essex, SS17 8EX, or the M.E. Action Campaign Group at PO Box 1126, London, W3 ORY.

Both the Association and the Action Campaign also publish regular newsletters, which are available to their members or to those on their mailing list.

The Christian approach

Since I have been treating post-viral syndrome, I have been amazed at the number of sufferers who are also Christians. My patient questionnaire asks people, before they have any contact with the clinic at all, to fill in their registration details; on it I ask them about their religion. More than half of the new patients I see are committed Christians.

I ask new patients if they knew that we were a Christian practice, and the answer is generally 'no'; gradually more people are being attracted to us that way, but for several years, almost all the patients who came to see us did not know that we were also Christian. The reason why what appears to be an epidemic of M.E. in the Christian population exists is a question of great interest to me. Almost all say that their faith has been greatly increased since contracting post-viral syndrome, and that the amount of time spent in thought, reflection and solitude has acutely increased their awareness of God's presence and His plan for their lives.

Praying for the sick

As a practice, we are all personally committed to praying for and with as many patients as will allow us to do so. We encourage every new patient to have an initial session of ministry to see how they feel about this form of treatment, and to follow it up if they wish. These treatment sessions are about an hour in length, during which they are able to discuss whatever feelings or emotions they may have about the treatment and the problems they are facing. Then one or two of the ministry team members will pray for the person.

I have had two patients who experienced dramatic healings within a matter of minutes after they have received prayer for their post-viral syndrome. However, eighty to ninety per cent of our patients get better with the whole treatment programme, and it is obviously difficult to say which component is doing which, but we believe we should continue praying for people. In some cases the prayer may heal, but in other cases in which the healing is not obvious, the person may feel encouraged by the fact that they have the attention of a number of committed people, and that someone feels that they are important enough to intervene on their behalf to ask God to heal them.

14 Live to recover

The primary rule in recovery from post-viral syndrome is to learn the difference between what you *think* you can do and what you'd *like* to do. No matter how severe or mild your illness is, the level of what you can do is definitely going to be less than you'd like.

In other words, we are talking about three different levels of activity:

Level 1: What you think you should be able to do
Level 2: What you can do without suffering a relapse
Level 3: The seventy-five per cent level, above which you cannot go if you want to get well

The challenge for recovery is to calculate level 2, at which you actually could function, and then to keep at seventy-five per cent of that level. This is probably the most important single step in recovering from post-viral syndrome. Most people realize that there is a compromise involved, but they think that it entails only doing what they can do, instead of what they want to do or should be able to do.

You then have to make a further compromise and do less than you're capable of if you are going to have any energy over to 'put in the bank' to aid your recovery.

For example, you may have a mild post-viral syndrome and think that you should be able to work full-time, socialize four or five nights of the week, clean your own house and do your own shopping. That is level 1. In fact, as you realize, you can in reality only work five days a week, and go out once or twice a week, even if you delegate your shopping. That is level 2. What you should be doing, level 3, is perhaps working four days a week, going out once or twice, and having help with the housework and shopping.

At the other end of the spectrum, if your illness is quite severe, you may find that all you can achieve is to get out of bed, have a bath and wash your hair, and for three afternoons a week sit down and talk to a friend. That then is your level 2. It is obviously very different from level 1, the amount that you feel that you should be able to do, and you have already been forced to make an enormous compromise. Unfortunately, if you are going to recover, you need to do even less than that for some time to come. You need to function at level 3, your seventy-five per cent level.

The recovery programme outlined in this book is going to involve many different approaches to conquering your illness. The first is changing your diet, and this has been discussed in chapters 9 and 10, on candida, and chapter 6 on food allergies.

Another aspect is a major improvement in your nutrition, and this we have discussed in chapters 7 and 8.

What we are looking at in this section is your lifestyle; this too will need to change considerably. Lifestyle includes your job, your relationships, your hobbies, your friends, your attitudes, and your leisure and exercise activities. No doubt you can think of many others, but these are certainly the most important ones.

Your job

Most people with post-viral syndrome will already have taken a considerable amount of time off work. If you are still at home but beginning to recover from your post-viral syndrome, you may well be thinking about what sort of occupation you could handle. The following points have to be taken into account; although they are probably common sense to many people without post-viral syndrome, they don't seem to be such common sense to those of us who have the driving mentality that so often succumbs to this illness. If you have only had the odd week off work and are struggling to hold down a job whilst trying to recover from post-viral syndrome, then you may be even less enthusiastic about what we have to tell you.

It is essential that you follow the rule outlined at the beginning of this chapter and do less than you think you can. So, for example, if you think you are well enough to go back to work two days a week, start by going back for only two mornings. Most people will have lived with the illness for some time, and therefore will get very excited when they start to recover, and push themselves too hard. It is then easy to become disillusioned at the slow rate at which they can return to normal, energetic society. Unless you want to plummet down with another relapse very soon, you really must follow the rule of doing less than you think you can.

The psychological stress of failed goals and failed achievements and hopes is enormous at this time. Failure can be damaging not only to your physical health, but also to your morale. As we have seen elsewhere, damage to your mental state can lead directly to damage to your immune system, and so the illness can enter another downward spiral.

Your relationship with your colleagues and your superiors is also very important at this time. If you delude yourself about your ability, stress yourself too far and suffer a relapse, then you will generate disillusionment about your ability to hold down the job. It is much better to make it very clear from the start that your functioning is going to be severely limited It is also important, of course, that you are open and honest about the problem from the very start, so that your employers can plan ahead, rather than being left in the lurch.

If you are seeing a doctor who knows something about post-viral syndrome, he or she will certainly be prepared to write you a letter explaining the circumstances to your employers or your school or university authorities. A little piece of paper such as this can be a powerful persuader in such circumstances.

It is also worthwhile speaking about the practical aspects of your work. For example, you should try and find employment that does not involve lengthy commuting every day, as this will exhaust you before you even arrive at your workplace. Ideally, the work should be sedentary, rather than requiring you to walk about. Similarly, try and find somewhere that does not involve climbing flights of stairs – a job on the ground floor, or one that is accessible by lift will make life easier for you, particularly if you have to move around in the building during the day. If it is at all possible, try and arrange to do some of your work at home, so that you can take days out of the office and conserve your energy. You will need to be set up with the necessaries for your work, be it a typewriter or a telephone or a sewing machine. Even better for you, of course, would be work that you can do without having to get out of bed. I (BD) still do a large amount of my administration, reading and writing from my home.

Finally, think about the crucial matter of holidays. Unless you take a considerable period of time off work in order to rest and recover your strength, you have much less chance of becoming well.

If you push your body to the limit, then as soon as any stress comes along, be it a physical one such as another illness, or an emotional one, then your life will crash. So if you are working full-time and think you are getting away with it, I would strongly recommend that you take stock of your circumstances, talk it through with your employers or colleagues, and reschedule your working life, if you can, so that you can take regular breaks. If at all possible, you should plan on eight or ten weeks of leave a year, broken up into several different holidays. Obviously some of this will have to be unpaid, but it is vital, as it will give you a far better chance to rest and recuperate than if you only had four or five weeks' holiday per year.

Exercise

Exercise has a number of benefits; it keeps your muscles in trim and your body functioning at its peak; it lets you mix in a gregarious group of people with whom you enjoy sharing a particular activity; and it gets you out into the fresh air and sunshine. In almost the entire population, it is an extremely therapeutic activity. However, even though we don't know exactly what is wrong in post-viral syndrome, the one clear thing we do know is that any exercise will make people worse. The only severe relapses I (BD) have ever seen in the cases of post-viral syndrome I've been treating were brought on by exercise.

The next problem is what constitutes exercise. For some people, exercise will be taking the dog for a long walk or playing some light form of sport. For others, exercise will be washing your hair and having a shower on the same day. Obviously, when your exercise tolerance is reduced to this last level, life becomes extremely difficult to cope with. In such a case, all we can tell you is that with resting beyond the level that you think you need, plus following the diets and regimes recommended in this book, and with the help of a sympathetic doctor, counsellor or therapist, you will eventually improve. You may not necessarily return to complete normality, but you will certainly be able to get considerably better. Never forget the rule we stated at the beginning of this chapter, that you need to do seventy-five per cent of what you think you can.

Hobbies

If you spend a large amount of your waking life working, you won't have a lot of space for hobbies. Nevertheless, you should still try and allocate some time for leisure activities which bring some colour and interest into your life. If, on the other hand, you do not go out to work, then you are going to need some activities that keep you challenged and feeling alive, but which do not involve a lot of physical exercise.

Please appreciate the need for leisure; don't spend your entire life doing those things which you regard as essential, and allow yourself no rest, recreation or relaxation. Once again, this problem is common in the driving type of personality that is so prone to post-viral syndrome. As such people realize that they are fifty per cent better, they immediately spend that fifty per cent of energy on keeping down a job and keeping their house organized, and completely forget to give themselves any time for rest or for simply being themselves. If this sounds like you, then please slow down! Think a little more about what you are doing, and if possible work a little less, allocate some of your responsibilities to somebody else, and be a little bit kinder to yourself.

Your good days are the dangerous ones

When you are ill and feeling exhausted, it is normal eventually to realize the fact, give in and go to bed. When you do this, you start to get better.

With post-viral syndrome, the most dangerous time for your health is when you think you are doing well, and especially when you are in a phase of improvement rather than a stable state. The reason is simple: when you are feeling good you are more likely to overdo it, and the overdoing is your undoing.

Many sufferers come to realize that their post-viral syndrome follows an up-and-down course (the medical term is 'relapsing and remitting'). This is usually quite close to what in mathematics is termed a sinusoidal curve (see first diagram overleaf).

When people are feeling ill, they go to bed, they rest, they take the steps that they know to be necessary, and soon they start to feel better (as shown in the second diagram overleaf).

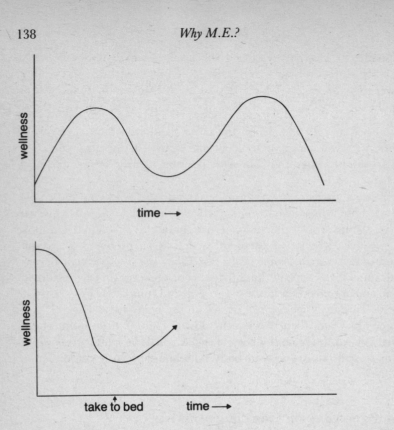

As they begin to recover, it seems that they are on the road back to health and are going to continue until they reach the normal level of wellbeing for which they have always been striving and hoping. As a result, like the horse bolting when it sees the stable door, they accelerate, and push themselves harder.

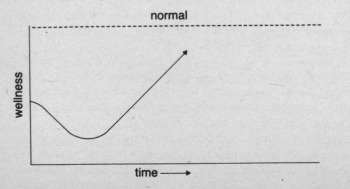

Sooner or later, they exceed the level at which they are really capable of functioning, which, as we pointed out earlier, is inevitably lower than the level at which they feel they *should* be functioning. As a result, they deplete their reserves of energy and they start to deteriorate. This may go on for quite some time.

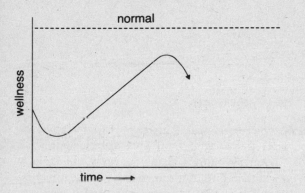

When things get bad again, everybody gives in. We give up, go to bed, rest and relax, and lo and behold, things start to improve.

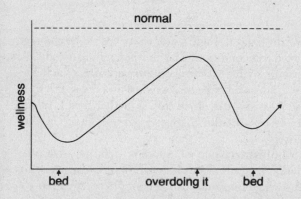

We are back on the same part of the roller coaster again. As things start to improve, we eventually reach the point where we think we are going to make it back to health again, and we start to push for it. So we overdo it again, and suffer yet another relapse.

This pattern is a major reason for appreciating the rule that we set out at the beginning of this chapter, of functioning at the seventy-five per cent level. When you accept this and realize that you are definitely

not a normal fit person, but need to live well within your limitations, is
when you will genuinely begin to recover.

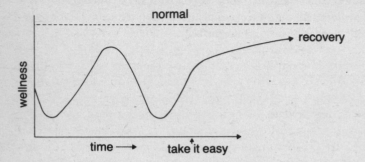

In this last diagram, you can see that if, instead of rapidly 'going for
it' as soon as you start to see your final goal approaching, you
deliberately calm down and slow down, then your body will actually
begin to recover. You will therefore continue to move in the direction
of health – but it will still be a long process, measured in terms of
months and years rather than weeks.

Attitudes

Your attitude can be the biggest single factor that needs to be changed
for you to recover from this condition. The characteristic attitude of a
large majority of people with post-viral syndrome is one of achievement and goal orientation, and of seeking reward and recognition. In
the section on personality, we discussed this in further detail. In this
section, we need to talk about the changes you must make in your
attitude in order to get better.

The driving, goal-oriented state of mind is definitely counterproductive to recovery. It needs to be changed, first, because it leads
you to keep busy the whole time and to expend more energy than you
can afford, and, second, because it exerts a psychological stress on
you, which puts a strain on your nervous system and therefore on your
immune system and your whole body.

Let us look first at the tendency to keep busy all the time. This may
be because you genuinely are a very active person with a very full life,
but it may also be a way of avoiding focusing on the problems in your
life – you keep your brain filled with minutiae so as not to focus on

what may be important but difficult or uncomfortable or painful. This is a tendency that needs to be changed, because it will lead you to exhaust yourself repeatedly and cause a relapse in your illness.

Only you can establish why you have this tendency, and indeed you may well need the help of an intelligent doctor or even a psychotherapist to analyse the problem.

You must learn to become happy and satisfied with a less than perfect existence. Try to get joy, pleasure and happiness out of what is going on around you. This may involve some changes in your attitude to other people and to your environment, and it may also involve making some changes in what *is* around you. Take a long hard look at your life, identify the fundamental changes that need to be made, and instead of constantly keeping busy by just changing the surface do something about the basics.

People who are constantly looking for achievements and are striving for goals are very often people whose own feeling of intrinsic self-worth is fairly low. It is essential for your recovery from post-viral syndrome that you begin to like yourself and become content with your own circumstances, your personality and your existence. You must learn to love yourself and not be driven by the need to change yourself, nor even the need to change others. Frustration at your inability to change things can lock you into a position of permanent stress, which will cause your immune system to become depressed and non-functioning. This can precipitate or worsen an illness such as post-viral syndrome.

For many people this is a very difficult process – far more difficult than any diet or vitamins we may recommend. If, after a long candid look at yourself, you suspect that this is part of your make-up, then we would strongly recommend that you see a therapist who is experienced in treating such problems. This should not be a matter of undergoing a lengthy course of analysis, but rather one of sorting out your day-to-day existence and helping you to start liking the you that really is, rather than the you that you are trying to be.

An essential part of developing a more contented lifestyle and overcoming the need to keep busy will be an alteration in the way you live your life at home. Try to make your living environment more peaceful and more relaxing. You can go some way towards this by simply changing the layout of your house. There are suggestions for doing this at the end of this chapter.

If there is somewhere comfortable in your office or workplace, you can curl up and rest at lunchtime – which will help you to last through the day.

Of course, only you can know exactly what will be right for your own environment, but there will definitely be a few simple changes that can help you to relax and be a little more peaceful. This will contribute substantially to your becoming more positive about the world and your own circumstances, and therefore about yourself.

It is also highly important that you appreciate that you *can* control the position in which you find yourself. You are not at the mercy of others, nor are you at the whim of circumstances. Many people with post-viral syndrome have a very circumstantial attitude to life; they feel that they are how they are because of the circumstances. We may not be able to wake up and decide to become Queen or Prime Minister, but we really do have the power to change our lives. It is only when we exercise that power and learn to make decisions, no matter how small they may be, that we actually come to have and to experience this control. Each decision that you make lets you know that you are in charge of your life. Each time that you take a decision about your life, you boost your morale, and therefore you boost your immune system and aid your recovery.

As well as feeling the victims of circumstance, many people with post-viral syndrome, or of the personality type that is particularly prone to it, suffer from low self-esteem. This naturally leads us to be controlled and manipulated by our perception of how other people see us. Of course, everybody apart from the victims of severe personality disorders or psychotic disorders is aware of and influenced by their sense of how others see them.

However, people with the striving personality type that is particularly prone to post-viral syndrome are also prone to the need constantly to prove themselves, both to themselves and to other people. If they fall victim to a disease such as post-viral syndrome, they therefore experience a strong sense of guilt and failure, and feel that they are devalued as individuals by the illness. It may well be necessary for you, if you are in this position, to work it through with a sensitive therapist.

Therapy can certainly help, but I would also like you to bear in mind that prayer can assist you in changing some of the deep-seated attitude problems you may have in your life. It can also enable you to change your own circumstances. Although there is certainly a lot we can do ourselves, I would recommend to anybody who feels the need for change, recognizes some of the points I have raised in this chapter, and realizes that there may be some changes needed in her life, should seriously consider asking God to help her with these changes.

The hardest lesson

The hardest lesson to learn when recovering from post-viral syndrome is that it never really goes away. Many people may burst into tears, shut the book and throw it away, or write me abusive letters for saying this, but if you've had the condition for more than about two years, then it doesn't completely go away.

I (BD) have seen over a thousand people with post-viral syndrome to date, and at the state of our medical knowledge so far, we have learnt to control it, to keep it completely at bay. People can be completely well so long as they live within certain limitations – but they are not cured. Cured means absolutely no illness, with absolutely no treatment, and absolutely no risk of recurrence. I don't think I have seen anyone cured of post-viral syndrome in the time I have been treating it.

Many people return to work and have happy and active lives, but if they start to exercise and get fit, have a very busy job and go abroad and catch dysentery then, when a number of things go wrong at once, they are at risk of succumbing again. My hope and prayer for the future is that we *will* find a way to cure this illness once and for all, but I must tell you that you need to learn to live with it – you can't just sit back, ignore it and wait for it to go, because it won't. Living with it means making changes.

On the brighter side (although you may not think there is a brighter side after that), if you can learn to live within your limitations and do not constantly push at the limits and overachieve, then you can have a very happy, fulfilled and challenging life.

Susie's story

My illness started two years ago when I had a flu-like illness from which I did not properly recover, due to a stressful following week. For one year I felt tired, with swollen glands, earaches and headaches.

I was told there was nothing wrong with me, although I felt all the time that I had some sort of recurrent virus. I am an immunologist working in a busy research lab at the Institute of Child Health. Money is short, and so for a long time we were understaffed. The pressure of work is also quite tremendous in this fast-moving field. After a period of completely overworking I became so unwell that I had to take time off work.

Due to my inability to cope with work, I suffered periods of tension which really didn't help my illness, and it became a vicious circle. I had used exercise to relieve tension, but I didn't have the energy any more and so I thought I'd try acupuncture. This has indeed proved helpful in relieving anxiety and generally making me feel more relaxed about life, which can only help the illness. It has no miracle cure, though, and my symptoms of M.E. actually got much worse as winter came on.

In February, when I was very unwell, I visited a herbalist who concocted a mixture for me to boost the immune system, cleanse the blood and lift any depression caused by the virus. She also advised me to take royal jelly and a clove of fresh garlic every day. This I took chopped up and swallowed down with food rather than chewed, with parsley to follow so I really didn't have bad breath.

There was a little improvement, although I was still unable to work, and it was not very dramatic.

In April I read some of Dr Dawes' articles and I started on a yeast-free diet, as I had convinced myself this could be the root of my problem. I had had an upset stomach for a few months and other symptoms. The sugar-free diet helped tremendously with energy levels, which are now much more even. It's so tempting to eat sweet things when you're tired. The yeast-free diet was excellent at cutting out junk food and most prepared foods with additives. Once you are used to it, it really isn't too difficult and it makes you think about what you eat.

After a holiday in May and being on the diet for a while, I was feeling much better and was able to return to work part-time. Holidays are like real battery charges for M.E. patients – provided the conditions are right: warm climate, not too long a distance to travel and at least some meals eaten out. It's a shame they can't be on prescription!

Amazingly, I joined a gym on coming back from holiday, for very light exercise to get me back into shape for working as my job is very physical. I coped with ten minutes on an exercise bike and some light weights machines twice a week for about six weeks, but it became all too much with the workload increasing. I went into relapse for several months when I couldn't even think of doing any exercise. I presume because I have not been desperately ill I have never actually been diagnosed as having M.E. and so was never advised against doing exercise until coming to Dr Dawes' clinic.

In June of 1988 I started attending Dr Dawes' clinic, seeing her assistant, Dr Collins. After losing a stone in weight, having been on a yeast-free diet for about three months, I lost a further half a stone on the low-carbohydrate diet. A lower body weight does require less energy to move around. The nystatin treatment caused nausea and headaches for the first few weeks, after which there was definitely improvement in the symptoms. The combination of supplements and intravenous vitamin C treatment has also helped me well on the way to recovery. I have yet to try the EPD treatment. I have only done the treatments for several months so far, but am excited about the future already.

These treatments are definitely of help to the recovery process, but I also believe that there is tremendous power in mind over body and that a positive attitude is essential for full recovery in this illness. I believe there is so much we can do by looking at our attitude to our illness and our whole lives.

I have recently decided to give up my job in conventional medicine research and follow my interests in alternative medicine in the hope that I may find a new career path. I now believe in a much more holistic approach to medicine, and the research that I was doing felt far too narrow.

Anthony's story

I am a designer-manufacturer, and up until 1980 I had forty-five craftsmen working in my workshop. I exported all over the world and had a large showroom in Sloane Street.

I was always in excellent health and very active – walking at least six miles a day prior to 1980, when I first began to notice how weak I was getting, especially when I had to be rescued from swimming in heavy surf on holiday. I had had PPP checks every year, which were negative, but I began to have numbness and pins and needles and heavy fatigue. I suddenly felt that premature old age had arrived in my mid-forties.

Then began endless visits to specialists all over London. I have a voluminous file resulting from these well-meaning doctors and their countless negative tests over a period of six years, at great expense. I finally read the *Observer* article on M.E. in 1986, which immediately gave me hope again – although by this time I had reduced my business very considerably and lost all my wonderful craftsmen. At least I now had a direction to start rebuilding again.

When I realized that I had M.E., I read all I could – joining the M.E. Association in England and also ANZME Society in New Zealand, immediately trying to define the cause, which I felt in my case (as in most patients) was multifactorial.

Firstly and most damaging, was the stress of running a large, complex business and being involved with various chemicals in my workshops; also a good dose of 'Rentokil' at home, which they omitted to warn one about; a three-month period of carbon-monoxide poisoning from a faulty gas boiler by courtesy of the gas board, which nearly finished me off; and recurrent viral infections.

After the pins and needles and numbness in my arms and legs, there followed a six-year period of many bizarre and unpleasant symptoms. I will try to name a few. Thank goodness they didn't all come at the same time!

Twitching and aching muscles; a continual sore throat affecting my speech; loss of memory; many neurological problems such as coordinating words; blurred vision; lightheadedness; vertigo; dizziness; susceptibility to excessive noise; endless migraines; hearing problems; chronic back and arm pains relieved only by cortisone injections; I was easily bruised and had tender spots all over the body, and had allergic rashes, mainly on my arms and legs; sometimes I also got very bad mouth ulcers and was extremely sensitive to hot and cold and sunburn effects even on a dull day.

There were, in addition, the dreadful depressions and panics, and even hallucinations resulting in thinking I was going mad and allowing my doctor to recommend a psychiatrist. I also had allergies to all the foods I had been eating, bloating, stomach and urination problems, sleep disturbances and, of course, the great aching and tiredness which sleep did not alleviate.

It was inevitable my business and social life suffered and so many people lost their jobs in my apathy.

However, the day I received my first pack of information from the M.E. Association I started to plan my recovery and eventually made an appointment with Dr Dawes, who started my long haul back to sanity and about an eighty-five per cent return to my old self – after about two years of treatment.

After various tests, I was placed on an anti-candida diet with a handful of vitamins to take three times a day and also nystatin, which I repeated for nine months before my head started to clear. I began my intravenous vitamin C treatments, which gave the old immune system a boost and, still following an ever-changing diet, avoiding many foods and drinking only mineral water, I slowly began to improve. I started on my EPD injections after several months and they eventually made me less allergic to most things. This treatment has continued over a period of two years, and I can now look forward to eating normally and drinking the occasional glass of white wine.

I am now feeling more optimistic about the future and rebuilding my business and social life again, after about eight years of unspeakable misery.

Lifestyle hints

I'd like to end this chapter by giving you a few helpful hints about how to organize your home. These are simple ways of making your life a little more comfortable and less demanding.

You should adapt your house to make it suitable for the kind of life you must have in order to recover. You need some comfortable sofas around to flop down on for ten minutes or an hour here and there during the day, to give your body a complete physical rest. Kitchen or dining chairs don't allow you to have a good rest; sitting bolt upright is not what your body needs.

Your kitchen should be really well stocked with the type of ingredients you need to cook, because you are not going to feel fit enough to pop out to the shop a couple of times a week when you realize you need something, as a fit and healthy person could do. Make sure you buy the ingredients you need for your diet in decent quantities so that you are not running out of them all the time. Not only can it be inconvenient and exhausting for you to have to go out, but the whole problem of shopping and cooking can come to depress you.

If you are on a highly specialized diet and you haven't got the necessary ingredients in your kitchen, you don't feel well enough to pop out to the shop, and you can't just ask the person next door if you could please borrow half a cup of buckwheat flour, then you can become very disillusioned and depressed about your isolation and helplessness. The way to prevent this is to be prepared, and keep organized.

By doing this you will also gain a positive feeling of satisfaction and control over your life, and this is as much a reinforcing spiral uphill as the downhill spiral that you have probably been experiencing up till now. The more you gain control over your life, the more you can feel self-confident, and the more this encourages your immune system to cope well with life and helps to maintain your ability to take in a good diet. And so the less ill you become, and the more confident you feel.

You should arrange your life so that you have to climb stairs as little as possible. Unless you are very ill, I am not advocating bringing your bedroom downstairs, although if you were choosing a new house, and there were two possibles, of which one was a bungalow, I would advise you to go for the bungalow without any hesitation. However, assuming you live in a house with your bedroom upstairs, then you need to organize things so that you climb those stairs as little as possible. The changes to your day can be very simple, such as having your bath or shower upstairs before going down to breakfast, rather than going down, making a drink or breakfast and then going upstairs again, only to have to come down again shortly afterwards. Very small differences such as this can minimize the physical effort required from you every day.

The next area to consider in this respect is the housework. As we have said before, it would be best if you could do no housework at all. If there is any way in which you can contract out to someone else as much as possible of the cleaning, cooking and general running of the house, then you really should do so. I know it is difficult to find people, and difficult to afford to have cleaners, but if your GP is sympathetic and understands that you're suffering from post-viral syndrome, he or she should be able to provide you with at least a few hours of home help via the social services. If, on the other hand, you are well enough to be working, even part-time, then one of the first things you should be doing with your income is having someone else to do your housework.

You should also choose a house that is low in maintenance. I am not advocating that you immediately put your house on the market and move, particularly since moving can be a thoroughly exhausting experience for somebody with post-viral syndrome. But we all do move for a variety of reasons, so when you are choosing somewhere to live please keep in mind that, although it may be lovely to have an enormous garden and a beautiful house, you may find your health benefits more if you choose something with lower maintenance. A flat in a newly purpose-built block would have the lowest maintenance of all, of course.

However, you may in this case find that you have landed inside a poisonous cubicle full of formaldehyde and other chemicals. If you are at all concerned about this, and remain so, having read our chapter on 'The world we live in' then I would suggest that you read Richard Mackarness's book *Chemical Victims*, as it is quite revealing about the alarming number of chemicals that are given off by modern building materials. In many ways the best place for someone with post-viral syndrome to live is somewhere at least ten years old, which hasn't recently been converted. It should not have lots of stairs, and if there is gardening to be done then there should be somebody else to do it, be it another member of the family, or just somebody coming round once in a while. When choosing an area in which to live, you may want to consider the proximity of relatives and friends who are likely to support you, as well as the travelling time to work for yourself and your partner, or to school for your children. Anything more than about fifteen minutes' travelling time each way adds very significantly to your burden for that day.

15　What about my family?

The M.E. victim is often not the only sufferer from the illness. The whole family can be affected by having a chronically sick person in the home, and in some cases they may even suffer from the disease themselves. In this chapter we look at the impact of M.E. on families, and the impact of families on M.E. They can help to make it better, just as much as they can help to make it worse.

Is it inherited?

We don't know exactly what kind of illness we are dealing with in post-viral syndrome. Although we have learnt how it affects people and what to do to help you get better, we don't completely understand the pathology of why people are ill. What we can say from our experience with a large number of patients is that there is no evidence that the illness itself is inherited. An inherited illness is one which is caused by something in the genetic material, the chromosomes. When somebody suffers from such an illness, we can predict that a certain percentage of their children will also be affected. Illnesses such as muscular dystrophy, Huntingdon's chorea and some other muscular and neurological diseases are obviously inherited. This is certainly not the case with post-viral syndrome.

You may, however, be thinking that it often seems to come in families, and why is this? The reason has more to do with family patterns of lifestyle and behaviour than to inherited problems. Although the illness is not inherited, there is certainly an inherited component in immune function. There is a vast range of strength and effectiveness in human immune capabilities, and it is obvious that some families are very strong and robust, while other families succumb to numerous illnesses.

Some interesting studies have shown that rats or mice which are fed a diet deficient in zinc develop a dysfunction of the immune system, and so do their offspring. If the deficiency is then corrected by giving zinc, it takes three generations before the immune dysfunction corrects itself! Although this is not an inherited disease in the genetic sense, it is an example of an inherited immune dysfunction. We believe that this is the kind of inherited problem we are dealing with in post-viral syndrome. There are a number of people who are especially susceptible to viral and other infections because the immune system that they have inherited is weakened.

The other important reason why M.E. runs in families has to do with behaviour patterns. Families tend to eat the same kind of diet and have the same kind of lifestyles. They go through times of stress together, and they have characteristic patterns relating to one another.

If one member of a family suffers from M.E., therefore, there are a number of environmental, nutritional and psychological reasons why other members of the family are likely to do so.

For example, you will have realized by reading the sections on diet and lifestyle, that these factors play a vital role in the development of and recovery from post-viral syndrome. If you come from a family that eats a high-sugar, high-carbohydrate diet with a good percentage of junk food, then it is likely that your whole family will be deficient in certain nutrients. As a result, you may all have immune systems that are weaker than those of a family that is eating a healthy nutritious diet.

If you come from a family that has an inherited defect in a minor metabolic pathway, this may cause you to have increased requirements for certain nutrients. If these requirements are not fulfilled, you will have a chronic metabolic malfunction and you will be more prone to a variety of illnesses than other people.

Families succumb to stresses together. If you are living in substandard accommodation, or have major financial difficulties or simply problems in coping with everyday existence, then you and your whole family are likely to be experiencing this together. Therefore, all of you suffer the effects of the stress, and may be more prone to infections as a result.

A number of research studies have shown that your risk of succumbing to a significant illness is strongly related to the number of points you score on a list of stress factors occurring in the previous twelve months. This is obviously of great relevance to some families who seem to have more than their share of post-viral syndrome sufferers; they are all likely to have similar and high stress scores.

Families also share patterns of behaviour and of relating to one another. If you come from a very goal-orientated family that is not good at showing warmth and affection, this is likely to affect your character make-up too, and make you (and your family) distinctly more likely to suffer from post-viral syndrome.

Can I catch it?

Of course you can catch it; obviously, if you are suffering from it you caught it from somewhere. However, it is very important to realize two points. First, it was not simply exposure to the virus or other organism that gave you M.E.; it was your own weakened defences. Second, you will not give it to everybody with whom you come into contact, as they will not share that weakness. If you are reading this book because you care about someone with post-viral syndrome, please take heart that once the disease is in its chronic stages, you are not at risk of catching it – as far as we know.

As we said in the previous section, we don't know exactly what M.E. is, so it is impossible to make hard-and-fast rules about the risk of being infected by it. From what we have seen in our medical practices, it is obvious that the disorder can be caused by a virus. However, the virus will only have this effect in certain susceptible people. In a large proportion of cases, we believe that it is one particular virus that is creating the problem. This is a member of the family of viruses which causes summer flu and stomach upsets, but in this case it affects vulnerable people in a much more unpleasant way. In many other cases, the viruses that cause glandular fever, chicken pox, mumps and many other diseases such as cytomegalovirus can apparently be the precipitating factor.

This view is not shared by some other researchers in the field who are pursuing the line that they have identified a single virus which is responsible for all cases. Whether or not they are justified in this claim, it seems clear that the virus will not have the effect of causing M.E. in somebody who is not already compromised, with their immune system not functioning properly. Put simply, it is very hard for a totally healthy person to get M.E.

Your GP may have told you that he has performed tests on your immune system, and those tests are normal, therefore your immune system is normal. We do not accept this; the available tests of immune functioning are limited and still unreliable, because the science of immunology is in its childhood still. For a doctor to make a claim such as this is comparable to saying to a patient 'because your blood tests are normal, those measles spots on your skin must be imaginary.' Unfortunately this is one of the commonest complaints that we hear every day in our practice. Traditional scientific medicine sometimes finds it very hard to admit to its shortcomings, or even to accept that it might have any at all.

For us, the message is clear: if you have post-viral syndrome, your immune system must be compromised. Someone else can certainly catch this virus from you, but unless their immune system is similarly compromised, they will not develop post-viral syndrome. They may catch flu, or diarrhoea, or whatever the virus is more used to causing.

It helps to think of this in terms of a balance between the virulence of the virus and the strength of your immunity. Virulence means how infectious and how damaging the virus is. A particularly virulent organism may cause post-viral syndrome in somebody who is only slightly under the weather. On the other hand, if you are particularly weak in your immune system, then a comparatively mild virus may cause you to develop post-viral syndrome, whereas in other people it would cause a much less serious illness, if anything at all.

This has been brought home to us very forcefully by the difference between patients in London and Scotland. Typical London post-viral syndrome sufferers are infected by a wide variety of viruses. They are all people whose immune system has taken a battering over a number of months before eventually giving in to the disease. This may have a lot to do with the more hectic lifestyle and the generally higher levels of pollution and environmental stress in London. Patients in Scotland, on the other hand, are typically fit, healthy and active until they are suddenly struck down by a specific virus, which has now been identified in many patients as a coxsackie B3 virus. This appears to be a virulent virus which has been responsible for a silent epidemic of M.E. in the Glasgow–Edinburgh area. This contrast is an example of the balance between the strength of the virus and the strength of your immune system which determines the outcome of the infection for you – a few days' flu or months and years of M.E.

Can I have children?

This is one of the questions I am most commonly asked by new women patients. The answer I give to them is that, according to our present knowledge, once they have followed the advice given in this book for at least twelve months there is absolutely no evidence that pregnancy and post-viral syndrome do not mix. Most women who are suffering from post-viral syndrome and become pregnant experience no worsening of their condition; moreover, all the babies I have seen born to women suffering from this disease have been normal, healthy babies.

As we have only been treating this condition for a few years, we have not yet been able to watch children born of mothers with post-viral syndrome grow up and have children of their own. Only when this happens will we be able to give you an absolute reassurance that everything will continue to be normal. We can only give you an interim report: so far, so good. In fact, many female M.E. sufferers who become pregnant find that their health actually improves during the pregnancy. - hormone changes.

However, the question about which you must think very seriously is whether, just because you are fit and healthy enough to carry a baby, you are also fit enough to look after a child for the next twenty years or more. Before embarking on a pregnancy, you need to give careful consideration to whether, in your state of health, you are capable of responding to the extra demands that a normal healthy child will place upon you.

If you have children already, you will know what I am talking about.

Obviously, a number of people will become pregnant in an accidental and unplanned manner, and under no circumstance would I recommend that having post-viral syndrome is grounds for abortion.

If your financial circumstances already enable you to have some help with your housework, and you are able to earn a reasonable living, and you feel you would be able to continue to do this and pay somebody to help to look after your children, then there is no reason why you should not go ahead. There will be demands placed on you, but they will be controllable and limited. However, if you are not fit enough to work and are feeling bored and lonely at home, and think that having a child would bring some purpose into your life, then I would strongly suggest that you spend a year or two following the treatments outlined in this book before you plan a family.

The demands of small children – sleepless nights, a twenty-four-hour-a-day commitment – are enough to drain any parent, let alone an M.E. sufferer. I am not suggesting that you don't have children at all, simply that you get yourself well enough to work and afford some help, even if you don't return to work, before you consider having children.

If reading all of this has not dissuaded you and you would like to become pregnant, then it is most important that you discuss the treatment you are receiving with the doctor who is supervising it. A number of the medications that we use in treating post-viral syndrome are not safe in pregnancy. Vitamin A and the amino acid tryptophan, for example, may both cause problems. A number of other treatments such as nystatin and EPD have not yet been thoroughly tested in pregnancy, and we cannot guarantee their safety for the unborn.

With children you already have, you can only do your best, love them as much as possible, and hope that one day they will understand the difficulties that you were experiencing while you were bringing them up, and why it is that Mummy or Daddy wasn't able to play football or go running with them like other children's parents. I think this is a very difficult problem for both you and your children, and I hope that you have sympathetic, supportive friends, neighbours or family who are able to do some of the more energetic things with your children that they need.

Relationships

Most people have at least one person in their lives to whom they are particularly close. They may be married, and as the majority of patients suffering from post-viral syndrome are women, most of the partners I am talking about will be husbands or boyfriends. The other relationships we need to look at are those of parents and close friends.

Partners

Whoever it may be that you have chosen to spend your life with, you expect that person to stay close to you and to help to fulfil your emotional and other needs while you offer them the same support. If the relationship was a good one before you became ill, then it is up to both of you to protect it as a valuable asset throughout your illness, and to look to a healthier future. Some people have a cavalier attitude to their relationship with their partner when they become ill. Although in these circumstances the relationship probably lasts during the illness, it may cause serious problems once the sufferer is recovering. If you are not married, you may be tempted to ignore this section. I would not recommend this, because what I have to say has important points for all sorts of relationships, both now and in your future.

Your marriage is of vital importance to you, and I believe it needs to be cared for. Keeping your marriage healthy while you recover is almost as important as recovering. I hope that through this book and any other treatments you may be having, you will return to health and discover that you have a marriage even happier and healthier than when you first fell ill.

However, many of you with post-viral syndrome will have come from marriages that were less than happy, less than supportive. This may, indeed, have been one of the reasons why you became ill. In this case, addressing the problems within the marriage itself with the help of a marriage guidance counsellor or a Christian counsellor trained in marital problems is the best way for you to work through your individual difficulties. Within the cover of this book, it is clearly impossible to discuss every kind of problem that may arise in a relationship, but there is one recurring pattern. This is that people find themselves in a marriage which is mildly unsatisfactory and creates a degree of stress for them, but they lack the confidence to attempt to change it. If this state of affairs is not dealt with, it will create greater problems in the future, possibly during the course of the illness, but more probably when you are recovering. I therefore strongly recommend that you try to bring about changes now, with the cooperation of your partner.

If you want your marriage to continue, and I hope you do, then it is also very important that you don't simply unload all the pressures of your illness on to your partner. If you have broken your leg in an accident and you are unable to walk for six weeks, it is normal to expect your wife or husband to take over your full set of domestic duties for that time. This seems perfectly within the bounds of reason in a marriage. If you have experienced it, though, you will realize that after a while the person who is doing the fetching and carrying will start to get bored. The unfortunate fact about post-viral syndrome is that it isn't for six weeks. It is a very long-term illness and recovery is slow. If you want your partner still to be there when you are better, the two of you need to look closely at the demands you place on one another.

I have asked a number of women patients to make a list of what they expect their husbands to do for them. The list includes:

Loving and caring
Providing a home
Providing enough money to keep the family supported
Doing domestic chores and maintenance around the house

On top of that they add activities such as:

Doing the shopping
Cleaning
Cooking all the meals
Doing all the ironing
Doing all the raising and disciplining of children
Providing a sympathetic ear for the frustrations of the person sitting at home trying to recover from M.E.
Being a sympathetic partner in a sexual relationship that may not to blooming at the moment

If you look thoughtfully at this list, you will realize that few people short of saints would be able to fulfil all these roles and to sustain them for months on end, as well as leading their own lives and holding down a job. What I recommend to most people is that you, the sufferer, decide that what you most want and need out of the relationship is the loving and caring. This, then, may have to be safeguarded at the expense of some of the other demands.

Many of the demands that we place on our partners can be spread around more widely and responsibility allocated to other people. As I mentioned earlier, if you can possibly afford it, a home help is very worthwhile. Although many people will say that they can't afford it, and many partners will say that they can cope with all the demands, my (BD) experience of treating many people with these problems is clear. If there is any way you can get outside help, either paid for by you or provided by the council, it is to be recommended. Having even part of the shopping, cooking and housework dealt with can seriously relieve the pressure that is felt by all members of the family of an M.E. sufferer.

Sympathetic friends or neighbours who can lend an ear or a shoulder to lean on are also extremely valuable. There are many people in the world who are willing to give you moral support over a cup of tea (even if it is herbal). This may make the difference between your partner coming home from work to an ear-bashing about how you feel, or to a happy smiling person asking how their day was. I would never suggest that you put on an unrealistically brave face, but you should seriously evaluate what you need from your partner and avoid overloading him or her, with possibly damaging results for the relationship.

There may also be problems with relationships that begin after you develop post-viral syndrome. Despite the hardships of the illness, it is possible to start a new relationship, particularly if you are on the road to recovery. There are many lovely, genuine, caring people in the world, and I hope that the person you are relating to is one of those; but just a short cautionary note – there are also a number of people who need to care.

They are different from the normal person who is happy to care. People who need to care have their own particular reasons for having a relationship with someone who is in a situation of need, and they can get a large degree of satisfaction and fulfilment out of caring for and looking after that person. Now, if you're not well, this may sound like heaven to you, but just think a little ahead. You want to recover, you want to get better, and one day you will. What will happen to that relationship when you are back to your outgoing, energetic self, and you are married to or in a permanent relationship with someone who needs to care for you in a very overt way? You are bound to feel differently, and the other person cannot be expected necessarily to change and adapt. You are unlikely to avoid serious problems with the relationship.

You also need your partner to be sympathetic to the fact that you generally don't feel as sexually inclined as you did before you got sick. If you want your partner to remain faithful, a sympathetic attitude on your part is essential. You must talk to each other about this; you must learn to communicate. If you overload your partner with excessive demands in this area, the stress may be more than he can maintain for months on end. He may then become ill himself, or shut himself off from the relationship, or even leave you on your own.

It is crucial that you and your partner are honest with one another, and if you feel that the relationship has no future, you must seek counselling for this and try to improve the position. If after this you still feel there is no future to it, then you must decide between you what action to take.

A problem that I have seen in a number of cases is that the M.E. sufferer feels that the relationship is to blame for her illness. She then feels very bitter about this, and exacts revenge on her partner by forcing him to look after her whilst she is sick. As soon as she is fit enough, she plans to punish him further by leaving. As well as being dishonest, this attitude is something that will definitely hinder her recovery. I hope that there are very few people reading this book who harbour these feelings.

It is crucial for you to be able to feel in control of your destiny and not put under stress by your circumstances. If your marriage is unhappy, you need to seek a remedy immediately. Do not carry on living with it as it is, especially if you have resentment and hate within you all the time. They will eat away at you and keep you ill.

Your parents

All our patterns of relationships are moulded by the way we relate to our parents as children, and they to us. Most of you with post-viral syndrome were probably brought up by parents who were encouraging you to achieve. You can't blame them for that; they brought you up to the best of their knowledge and ability. In the forties, fifties and sixties, goal-orientation and rewards for desired behaviour were the way parents were encouraged to raise their children. This has produced a generation of young adults who are very ambitious but do not set a high value on their own self-worth. They as a generation were rewarded for good behaviour rather than for just being themselves, and they still feel that good behaviour and achievement are expected of them.

If your parents do relate to you in this way, then you are probably going to find them difficult during the process of recovery. You need to recognize that they are likely to fall into one of two groups. They may try and encourage you to achieve, saying such things as, 'I'm sure you are well enough to get back to work now, why don't you just try.' This will be done in a loving and caring way, but without real understanding of the position you are in. They may always be gently encouraging you to overdo it, in effect. You have to resist this. Only you can finally judge the amount of energy that you can afford to spend on life, and still have some left to use in recovery.

You may be able to resist by discussing the problem with them and talking it through, but you may need to see less of them and put some distance between you and them.

The other problem you may encounter is similar to that which we discussed earlier, regarding partners who 'need to care'. Many parents need a degree of control over their adult offspring and involvement in their children's lives. As long as the child remains a child, life is wonderful and they will be exemplary parents in order to keep the child near them, and dependent on them.

Eventually, however, we all grow up and leave our parents, and if they fall into this last category they will find it more difficult than most to cope with this. They may try and keep the apron strings quite active, even though you physically left home long ago and have been completely self-sufficient for years. When you fall victim to post-viral syndrome, although parents may on one level find it abhorrent that their child is suffering from this disease, on another level they find that the simplest response pattern is to revert to the old one of looking after you completely, and having you dependent on them. If your parents fit this category they are acting not only out of love, care and concern for you, but also from a deep intrinsic need within them to feel needed, which drives them to mollycoddle you.

Neither of my parents fitted this category at all, and I must say that for the first few years that I was sick, I was quite envious of friends also suffering from the condition who seemed to be able to retreat to a wonderful home environment and have their every whim catered for. However, having now seen many, many more people with this condition, I realize how incredibly insidious this situation is. I lived for a while with one friend whose parents fitted this category absolutely, and I suspect that she will never recover unless she eventually realizes that her parents' need to look after her is part of what is keeping her ill.

The central message of all of this should by now be clear to you: we need to feel responsible for and in control of our own destiny, even if that destiny consists merely of what time to take a bath and what time to have lunch. When we are in control and able to make the decisions about where our life is going, then gradually those decisions become bigger and bigger, and as they do it is possible for us to become healthier and healthier.

I would very strongly advocate that you do not allow yourself to fall into this position of becoming a child again and being looked after, no matter how comfortable it may be in the short term.

If your parents really do love you and really do want you to get better, then by all means ask them to care for you while you are acutely ill; but as soon as you are well enough to be living on your own again, you must break out. Of course you can ask them for some financial help in looking after yourself, or for more support from a distance, but do not revert to the parent/child relationship, which can become harder and harder to break free from.

Having said this, I must add that I have seen a number of perfectly happy, supportive families with one member suffering from post-viral syndrome. Please don't think that your parents and family can only fall into one or other of the two groups I've described. These are simply two patterns of response by relatives that I have seen often and feel are worthy of discussion. If, on the other hand, you have an excellent, healthy relationship with your parents, then good for you and good for them. Please look after it.

Friends

Friends can be a problem for the M.E. sufferer. The relationships are less intense than those with your partner or your parents, and are naturally far less committed. Friends often feel that they can come and go like the wind.

They take no vows of 'for better, for worse, in sickness and in health', and as many of you will have found out, in sickness they just aren't there. It may be true that 'a friend in need is a friend indeed', but many of you may have discovered that all your friends have turned out to be fair-weather friends. If you are feeling sad, lonely and rejected because people who you thought were close friends have left you since you became ill, please don't feel you are alone. This is one of the unfortunate side effects of this illness and we have almost all had to cope with it.

Most of your friends will fall into two categories. They will either be outgoing, driving people, with goal-orientated lives, as you have very probably been – sharing, in fact, the very tendencies which helped you to become ill. If so, then they will have difficulty appreciating how ill you are. They may say to you, 'Come on, you must be able to do a little bit, it will be good for you,' or, 'It will be good for you to go out, it'll brighten you up.' With the best will in the world, they will be forever encouraging you to overdo things, and they will therefore definitely hinder rather than help your recovery.

While my secretary was typing this manuscript for me, she said in exasperation at one stage how tedious and how boring and wet she found my advice, and asked me why I was encouraging patients to give in to themselves so much. This is exactly the response that I am describing. Needless to say, we had a long talk.

Clearly, it is better for me to have a secretary who is driving and ambitious, but if your friends are driving and ambitious too, they will never understand the extent to which you need to give in to this condition.

The other major group of friends, and those with whom you will probably find that you make the best friendships while you are suffering from M.E., are the quieter, less energetic people who are much less aggressive in their lifestyles and their approach to the world. Such people can be far more helpful to your recovery, as they are not going to push you. On the other hand, they in turn will fail completely to understand why, every time you get part-way better, you get out there and 'go for it' again; they are simply not possessed with the same driving force that you probably are.

In short, knowing the problems that most people have had during the course of this illness with keeping their friends, the best advice that I can give you is that if you have a few friends who are standing by you, then value them and treat them well. They are an extremely important asset to you.

16 Getting away from it all

Why go?

The reasons for getting away from this country are many: the stress of our city lifestyles, the moist damp climate, the enormous amount of pollution in our air and food, the need for relaxation and a boost to our morale. These are all valid reasons for trying to spend some of your time in a healthier environment.

When the illness is at its worst, and you are wholly or partly bedridden, it may be extremely hard for you to go on any sort of holiday. After you have followed a treatment programme, such as the one described in this book, for some time, and are starting to feel significantly better, the picture changes. Holidays become a viable proposition, and they can also become an important part of your treatment regime.

The people for whom this is easiest are obviously those who were in regular full-time employment and were lucky enough to be covered by some sort of health insurance. Unfortunately, for the majority of sufferers on supplementary benefit or sickness benefit, this is not so simple.

As I have already said, for those of you who are managing to work, I strongly recommend, if you have a cooperative employer or are able to choose your own working regime, that you attempt to negotiate an arrangement whereby you can have between eight and twelve weeks' holiday a year. The purpose of this is not to allow you to become a world traveller, but to allow you the extra time to organize your life, rest, and catch up on the sleep that the average person does not seem to need.

When to go

There are very few times when one really should not take a holiday, but if you are suffering from post-viral syndrome, you should avoid going to sunny summer places in July, August and September. These are the times when delays are far more likely and airports and resorts are crowded. You are less likely to get individual attention for your dietary and any other special requirements. The best times for going away, I would suggest, are spring and autumn. April and May are ideal because your body is drained and run-down from the long winter.

In October or even November moulds are particularly prevalent in the British atmosphere, and if you are mould sensitive, as so many patients with post-viral syndrome are, then this is a good time for a change of scene.

On the other hand, many post-viral syndrome sufferers find that their illness varies with the seasons, and that they have a particularly low period in January, February and March. Their fatigue is worse, their moods are worse, they crave carbohydrates more and gain weight, and they are more prone to infections – and often to allergies too, particularly chemical sensitivities. In general, everything seems to be grinding to a halt. This pattern is very reminiscent of seasonal affective disorder, and in fact a lot of the patients we see appear to have a 'seasonal physical disorder', which also has its worst period in the first three months of the year. If this sounds like you, then it will be highly therapeutic for your immune system and your whole body to have an input of sunshine at this time.

As few people can afford to go abroad more than once a year – if that – you should decide which time would be particularly beneficial for you.

Where to go

There are a number of places that make excellent holiday destinations for M.E. patients.

Lakes and mountains

Holidays in lakes and mountains can be brilliant – if you are staying in a hotel or bed-and-breakfast with a beautiful view over a lake, and you can take a short wander to sit on a sunny terrace watching the water and soaking up the scenery. However, this type of holiday is quite inappropriate if you are with a group of people who are planning on climbing mountains or hiking for several days. It is extremely difficult to be on holiday with people when they are planning on doing a considerable amount of activity and you are unable to be with them and see them if you do not join them in these activities.

The benefit of high mountain holidays is quite incalculable. I certainly find that my health improves dramatically whenever I am in a mountainous environment such as the Alps.

The reasons for this, I would say, are probably related to the exhilarating environment, beautiful scenery, absence of pollution, lack of humidity and therefore mould, and possibly the high level of negative ions. In fact, the Alps, and high mountains in general, have always been recognized as having therapeutic properties. They were the site for a number of sanatoria established to treat patients with tuberculosis. The major reason for this seems to have been the opportunity to soak up large doses of sunlight, which at high altitudes has a significantly higher content of ultraviolet light, but without the exhausting effect of high heat levels.

The Mediterranean

The Mediterranean is certainly the most popular holiday destination for Britons travelling abroad, and I would thoroughly recommend a holiday there to anyone suffering from post-viral syndrome. Greece, Turkey and the Portuguese Algarve are all excellent places for a relaxing sunny holiday to top up your sunlight levels and stimulate your immune system.

Of the countries around the Mediterranean, my personal favourite would certainly be Greece. Greek food combines exceedingly well with an anti-candida diet, the Greeks are a friendly and hospitable nation and, as they are members of the EEC, one feels a certain degree of security should things go wrong. I felt more vulnerable in Turkey, in the sense of health care and follow-up should anything unfortunate occur, but apart from that little uncertainty Turkey is an excellent destination for a restful holiday.

I would avoid Italy and France, because the culture is more developed and the people are less co-operative about providing the kind of diet you need. Also, you may find it very hard, except in the more remote areas, to <u>avoid pollution</u>. Similarly, I would not go to Spain for a relaxing holiday in the sun, because half the rest of the country is doing so and unless you go to some exclusive resort you are likely to be crowded, bustled, and unable to find the individual service you probably need to cope with your problems.

Portugal, on the other hand, in my experience has been far less plagued by this. Hotel and restaurant staff seem more co-operative than in Spain, and it does seem to be slightly less crowded. It is also excellent for villa-type holidays, where you can do your own cooking and control your own diet without stress.

I would not recommend the southern (African) coast of the Mediterranean for patients with post-viral syndrome, as the incidence of 'tummy bugs' is much higher, and the general level of health care much lower, than in the north and eastern Mediterranean, so that you may find you are in a more severe predicament after your holiday than before.

Winter sunshine

Winter sunshine is something I would strongly recommend for all those who can possibly afford to get away and break the depressing long winter in this country. Destinations such as the Caribbean and Florida are obviously expensive, but can be less so than you think if you only go for a week or ten days, and stay in a simple self-catering apartment. My personal choice would be Barbados in the Caribbean, although Florida can also be the setting for a very pleasant winter sunshine holiday. However, I would not recommend holidays in America in general, as obviously they fulfil very few of the requirements of a holiday for an M.E. sufferer. The pollution level is high, and there are so many exciting things to do and see that you'll be tempted not just to sit and relax.

Finally, wherever you go, avoid pollution and hills. It is amazing how many people choose to take their holidays in polluted areas where they are going to be imprisoned in their hotels because the surrounding countryside is quite unsuitable for them to be able to venture out.

Where not to go

Just as crucial as deciding the holiday you should go on, is to avoid the sort of holiday you shouldn't. If you are considerably disabled and barely able to get out of bed, you are unlikely to make the mistake of being over-optimistic and overstretching yourself.

However, those of us who are working with our M.E. are far more prone to biting off more than we can chew in terms of ambitious holidays.

The first kind of holiday to avoid is a touring holiday, particularly with other people who don't have M.E. A holiday driving, inter-railing or on a bus tour may seem quite relaxing to some people, and can certainly be a very enjoyable holiday. But to have to be up at a certain time every day to fit in with other people, not to be able to rest when you want to or to take life at your own pace will soon make you realize how you are functioning. It may only be at a ten per cent slower pace than those around you, which is not noticeable in your day-to-day existence. Come holiday time, your friends or family are all capable of a 7 A.M. start, and of driving through well into the evening, and then getting up and doing the same thing the next day – but you are obviously not. This type of stress could precipitate a serious relapse.

The second kind of holiday to avoid is one which requires you to have injections before you go. All forms of immunization seem to make people with post-viral syndrome worse. (However, if you need a tetanus injection because you trod on a rusty nail, then clearly you must have your tetanus injection and take the chance that it may precipitate a minor relapse of M.E.)

The other places to avoid are the ones from which almost everybody you know comes back ill. Some countries are renowned for having different bugs which affect our intestines in different ways from the ones encountered at home. You can be sure that if you are suffering from M.E. and get a tummy bug, it will be the end of your holiday.

The other easy way to ruin your trip is with jet lag. You should avoid long-haul flights where jet lag is going to be a problem, unless you are going for a considerable length of time. For going to Australia or New Zealand, you would need to allow yourself about five days at each end when you are not committed to any form of activity, to recover from your jet lag.

The idea of spending five days in bed when you arrive may be daunting; even more important is the five days in bed when you return. M.E. sufferers are far less capable of adapting to jet lag than other people and, if you try to ignore it and battle on, you may well precipitate a relapse.

For travelling to the East Coast of America and the Caribbean, allow yourself two or three days either side to recover from the jet lag. Travelling to the Middle East, allow two days to recover, and for the Far East, five days again.

There are numerous diets and regimes for coping with jet lag, and I've probably tried every one of them, usually in conjunction with friends who are travelling on the same flights. Although these regimes, on the whole, work for my friends, they don't seem effective for people with post-viral syndrome, and I think the only solution is to schedule time to do nothing except recover.

Another kind of holiday to avoid is one that involves a lot of walking. When someone says, 'Let's go for a romantic weekend in Paris,' you may each be conjuring up completely different ideas. To you a romantic weekend may be breakfast in bed each morning shortly before midday, followed by sitting at a street corner café for half the afternoon, and then a short sightseeing ride in a taxi, and then a nice restaurant for dinner. Your companion may have an entirely different idea and be thinking that you can visit four galleries before lunch, and five different major department stores and shopping streets before going to the theatre or opera in the evening. Both ideas make great holidays, but if you are suffering from post-viral syndrome, the latter holiday would see you back in bed fairly smartly.

Being realistic in your choice of city holidays is important. There is no reason why a person with post-viral syndrome can't visit a city and see its galleries, shops and museums, but you have to keep your walking to a minimum, use taxis as much as possible, and avoid stairs wherever you can. This may all sound like common sense, but hardly a day goes by in my office without someone ringing up in tears because they went to Rome and couldn't cope, or were made so ill by the yellow-fever injection that they had to cancel their holiday.

You should also avoid holidays in noisy places. This, like most of the advice in this book, is going to seem a statement of the obvious, but in a glossy brochure a hotel with a panoramic view of a picturesque bay may seem everything you've been looking for, until you realize that it is next to the resort's largest disco.

If you are not suffering from post-viral syndrome, this is only likely to annoy you, not to precipitate a major illness. However, spending a week without getting a decent night's sleep while suffering from M.E. may mean that you spend the next three months in bed. Before booking any holiday, ask some searching questions, and I would very strongly recommend that you send the travel agents a letter stating your problems and asking for a signed copy of their reply before you pay for your holiday.

What type of holiday?

The only feasible holiday for people with post-viral syndrome is a single-destination holiday. You have to weigh the stress of travel against the enjoyment gained from it, and this only balances in your favour if you go to a single place.

The advantages of flying on scheduled flights are considerable. There are fewer delays than on charter flights, in-flight comfort is better, and the extent to which the airline is prepared to cater for your particular needs, be it special diet or assistance at the airport, is also greater. Besides, when you check in for a scheduled flight, there are likely to be five or six check-in desks and a short queue. For a charter flight there will be one or two check-in desks and maybe two hundred and fifty people in front of you. Queuing for twenty minutes or an hour in a crowded airport is not likely to start your holiday off on the best foot.

For people with M.E. who are travelling with people without M.E. the best holidays are those with a single destination and a number of sporting activities available, so that the 'fit' people do not feel restrained by the problems of the person with M.E. On such a holiday it is quite acceptable to sit by the pool sipping mineral water and doing absolutely nothing for two weeks except soaking up the sun, while your companions spend the day windsurfing and waterskiing, paragliding and scubadiving, and meet you for breakfast, lunch and supper – so no one feels left out.

What about skiing?

Skiing holidays can be brilliant, and if you're addicted to them there is no reason not to go, unless you really can't stop yourself from doing too much exercise.

What is too much exercise? We said in chapter 14 you need to do about three-quarters of what you think you can do, which is different from what you think you ought to be able to do. If it is an effort for you to climb a single flight of stairs, then on a winter holiday you should only be riding the cable cars and meeting your friends for the odd drink at mountain restaurants.

If your M.E. is under control and you are doing well on the treatment programme, working five days a week and quite able to cope with a normal life, but not quite up to the pace of your friends, then a winter holiday where you maybe do a couple of hours' skiing a day is probably within your reach. Again, you need to do a lot less than you think you can, and not to bite off more than you can chew. My tolerance to skiing probably comes because I am such an addict, and if you aren't an addict it's a sport to avoid.

If you had been skiing for many years before you got post-viral syndrome, and your skiing standard is good, then by going back a grade or two in the runs you take on, a few hours' skiing can be no more taxing than just standing still, and considerably more enjoyable as you glide gently down blue and green, and the occasional red run.

Under absolutely no circumstances, no matter how well-controlled your illness, should you start learning to ski if you are suffering from post-viral syndrome. This is an absolutely exhausting experience even for the fit, and for M.E. sufferers it is out of the question.

If I have put you off skiing but you still need a winter break, then lying on a beach somewhere in the sunshine would be by far the most advisable holiday.

What type of hotel or apartment?

Hotels are often easier for people with disabilities, in that they are usually well placed for the object of your trip, be it beach or city, and they are well staffed. You can virtually have a holiday without having to lift a finger.

Before you book a hotel, get its telephone number, ring up and speak to the staff. If you don't feel that they are cooperative, move on and look for a different hotel. If staff are not cooperative before you've booked in, they are very unlikely to be so afterwards.

Hotel position is equally important. If you've gone to soak up the sun, then the hotel needs to be on the beach, preferably with its own swimming pool.

If you have gone to stay with friends while they are skiing, and you're doing a bit of skiing and meeting them in restaurants, then location is even more important. Skiing terrain is quite primitive for the average person with M.E.

Your hotel needs to be close to the lift system, well placed for any buses you may want to catch or whatever view you have come to look at. You do not want to be stuck in your hotel room for the whole holiday because you are unable to make the half-mile walk uphill to the bus stop. These things are worth finding out beforehand.

One of the most crucial things in a hotel holiday is that the chef speaks English. Telephone the hotel and ask to speak to the chef at a quiet time of the day; explain to him that you're coming to stay and that you have some special dietary requirements, and see what sort of reception you get. Not many chefs are going to be too excited at having to cook special diets, but see if you can get some cooperation. You can, of course, offer to bring any special ingredients with you.

Better still, write to the hotel first, then about ten days later phone and speak to the chef; see whether he has had your letter and how he feels about it, rather than suddenly putting him on the spot at what might be an extremely inconvenient time.

Another question well worth asking about the hotel is whether you can actually see anything from your bedroom. Many hotels have a good view but you need to be standing up and looking out of the window to see it. If you are reasonably debilitated by your post-viral syndrome, and are going on a holiday where you might be spending at least half your day in bed, then probably the most important thing to choose is a hotel where you can actually see the mountains or the sea from your window whilst sitting in bed.

Something else I would very strongly advise against is a meal-plan or half-board system. If you go into a restaurant seating five hundred people and expect the chef to adapt the meal plan to you, you are unlikely to have much success. It is worth paying a little bit more to eat in an à la carte restaurant, where the staff are able to deal with you on a one-to-one basis and you are much more likely to get the diet you need.

I'm sure people with post-viral syndrome would not forget to ask the hotel this, but do check that it has a lift. Many hotels think nothing of asking their clients to walk up five flights of stairs to their bedroom.

One thing to check – I speak from bitter experience – is that they will not put you in a room on top of the disco or immediately next to where the band plays during dinner. Try to get a commitment on this in writing.

My final advice on the hotel is to check with the management that you can actually open the windows. Many people with post-viral syndrome are chemically sensitive. Most are not overwhelmingly so, but lock yourself in a hermetically sealed formaldehyde-lined box and you will soon find out exactly how sensitive you are. Opening a window will usually solve the problem. If you can't, you may find that you have difficulty sleeping, and after a time, your M.E. could become considerably worse.

Apartments

Much of what I have said can apply equally to apartments, and the chief advantage of an apartment over a hotel is that you can do your own cooking, and therefore control your diet much more. But because of that element of control, you are doing more work, and the holiday is therefore less relaxing; so you have to judge the balance for yourself.

Your apartment should be near to the supermarket and shops, and if you can have a deal from your travel agent whereby the apartment includes a rented car, that is obviously far more suitable as it reduces the amount of shopping to be carried by hand.

Again, try and establish that the bedroom has some sort of view. Apartment buildings are less likely to have lifts, so be specific about obtaining a ground- or first-floor apartment – and again, try and get it in writing. Check with the travel agent that the apartment is not too near a disco that will go on playing music across the rooftops till 3 or 4 A.M. every night.

At the airport

The hectic disorganization that tends to occur at airports can be enough to spoil your holiday completely. As a first plan of attack, enlist the help of one or two understanding friends. If you are suffering from post-viral syndrome, this is something you have to get fairly good at doing. It's difficult to ask friends to do something for you that you know they don't even enjoy doing for themselves, but if it's possible, get a friend to pick up your bags, tickets and passport half an hour before you leave home, and to go and queue for you at check-in. That way you are not sitting around – or, more to the point, standing around – in the airport for quite so long.

If you meet them at a prearranged place in the airport, it can reduce the amount of hassle you have to go through. You should notify the airline in advance if you have particular meal requirements – but I would not rely on them to remember. Most often they do, but when they don't you can guarantee that yours will be the flight that is delayed for seven hours, and the airport that took you three hours to get to from home, so you should take food for about twenty-four hours with you, in order to cope with any kind of airport contingency.

You can buy mineral water almost anywhere in the world, so you don't need to carry large volumes of liquid with you, but I would suggest you take some snacks, and in particular protein, sufficient for two or three meals, so that should everything go wrong at once, and you are unable to buy anything suitable at the airport, at least you will not collapse from hypoglycaemia.

The last point to remember at the airport is that you can go as a disabled passenger and request a wheelchair if you want. Obviously, people suffering from M.E. are not often seriously disabled, but if it doesn't embarrass you too much to feel conspicuous, this can certainly be a way to avoid all the walking, bag-carrying and queuing that is required at an airport.

Insurance

Before you go on holiday, check with your GP that, in his or her opinion, you are fit to go, because if you have done that, you have covered yourself in case any deterioration in your health causes you to cancel. Should anyone then query that you are suffering from a chronic illness, you can honestly say that you have booked the holiday on medical advice that you were fit enough to go.

Enjoy yourself and have a good time.

Resource File

British Society for Nutritional Medicine
Secretary: Dr P. J. Kingsley
72 Main Street
Osgathorpe
Leicestershire

British Society for Allergy and Environmental Medicine
Secretary: Mrs Ina Mansell
'Acorns'
Romsey Road
Cadnam
Hampshire

✗ Myalgic Encephalomyelitis Association
Secretary: Mrs Searles
P.O. Box 8
Stanford-le-Hope
Essex
SS17 8EX

✗ M.E. Action Campaign
Secretary: Mr Martin Lev
P.O. Box 1126
LONDON
W3 0RY

Action Against Allergy
Secretary: Mrs A. Nathan-Hill
43 The Downs
LONDON SW20

Books

Candida Albicans – Leon Chaitow, Thorsons Publishers Ltd, 1985.
Not All In The Mind – Dr R. Mackarness, Pan Books Ltd, 1976.
The Yeast Connection – Dr William Crook, Biosocial Publications Europe, 1983.
The Food Allergy Plan – Dr Keith Mumby, Unwin, 1985.
Day Light Robbery – Dr D. Downing, Arrow Books, 1988.

Food Suppliers

Foodwatch International Ltd – Butts Pond Industrial Estate, Sturminster Newton, Dorset, DT10 1AZ.
Victoria's Wholefoods Delivery Service – Telephone 01-461 3647

Supplements

Lamberts Dietary Products Ltd – 1 Lamberts Road, Tunbridge Wells, Kent, TN2 3EQ
Thorne Research Inc. – 986 Industry Drive, Seattle, Washington 98188.
Klaire Laboratories – 126 Acomb Road, York, YO2 4EY.

Index